THE BADASS BODY DIET

THE BADASS BODY DIET

The Breakthrough Diet and Workout for a Tight Booty, Sexy Abs, and Lean Legs

CHRISTMAS ABBOTT

WITH MAGGIE GREENWOOD-ROBINSON

wm

WILLIAM MORROW
An Imprint of HarperCollinsPublishers

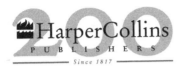

HarperCollins books may be purchased for educational, business, or sales promotional use. For information please e-mail the Special Markets Department at SPsales@harpercollins.com.

A hardcover edition of this book was published in 2015 by William Morrow, an imprint of HarperCollins Publishers.

FIRST WILLIAM MORROW PAPERBACK EDITION PUBLISHED 2017.

Designed by Lisa Stokes

Photography by Josh Homes Photography

Library of Congress Cataloging-in-Publication Data has been applied for.

ISBN 978-0-06-239096-7

17 18 19 20 21 DIX/LSC 10 9 8 7 6 5 4 3 2 1

For my mother, Barbara

From you I inherited my great tenacity for loving life, embracing what I believed in, and never accepting anything less than what I wanted no matter what hand I was dealt. Your strength and passion are unmatched in this world. You will always be my hero and purest inspiration.

Contents

PART 4: LIVING THE BADASS LIFESTYLE

Acknowledgments

A simple *thank-you* cannot convey the gratitude I have for the collective team that helped me in my journey that led me to this place today. This book wouldn't be possible without them:

My agents, Abbey MacDonald and Steve Troha, who are more than agents—they're warriors! Their belief in my work amazes me.

My coauthor, Maggie Greenwood-Robinson, was incredible to work with. Her creativity is priceless!

The incredible team at William Morrow/HarperCollins who saw the potential in this book, and in me.

All of the fans who wrote to me asking for advice and trusting in my words. Keep the course and stay relentless!

Most of all, my mother, who always believed in me no matter where I was in life.

Body Booty-ful

ALL DAY LONG, I hear from women who crave a round, neat booty that looks fabulous in and out of clothes, but don't know how to get it. A lot of them even go for crazy quick fixes, like padded pants or silicone undies designed to push up the butt like a padded bra pushes up boobs, and some even have cosmetic surgery to get a butt lift.

Are you one of these women? You don't have to step forward or raise your hand, but are you obsessing over your lower body? Would you rip the bottoms out of some old jeans if you tried to wriggle into them? Are you hiding your lower body under long black skirts? Has another trip to the clothing store ended in frustration and fury at being unable to find anything that fits?

Can you relate? I can! I get your frustration. We women tend to carry more fat in our booty than men do. Sure, this extra wad of fat is great for baby making, but it's horrible for bikini wearing—or for catching an eye for baby making. We want so badly to change our hips and buttocks, and overall body. In fact, we're obsessed with the idea.

We can do it easily, naturally while having FUN, I say.

For too long, experts have told us that having a large booty and soft lower body *protects* a woman's health. Totally not true! For the first time in book form, I'm going to rip through that myth and reveal why firming up your butt will not only give you a sexy body, it will also give you a stronger heart, more functional mobility, and a lot of other benefits that no one has talked about until now. I've decoded the female anatomy and figured out how we can conquer that defiant fat on our butts, and in doing so, achieve strength, power, and sexy curves from head to toe. Oh, and did I mention confidence?

No fitness book has adequately addressed what to do about a saggy, flat, flabby butt—which is why I wanted to write my first book on this often-neglected topic. For many years now, I feel that the fitness world has been overly focused on tummies. There's a flood of books out there about how to eat and exercise for flat abs. I'm so sick of all the "flat belly" programs out there. They just create skinny-fat girls instead of strong toned bodies, and not much else. When you focus on your booty, the rest of your body—including your belly—gets thin and fit too.

Oh, and besides the fixation on bellies, there's the boob thing. Talk about sensory overload. Guys have been so overexposed to boobs, in girlie magazines, music videos, and busty tight tops, that breasts have lost their special fascination. But the butt . . . ah, it's much sexier. And guess what? It was a sexual turn-on in ancient times, long before breasts ever were. Anthropologists—scientists who study old bones—will tell you that when people lived in caves, humans mated the way all other mammals still do—from the rear. That's right. The sexiest chicks back then were those with the nicest butts.

Today, we've come full circle: Men's eyes are back on the original "breast," the butt. In fact, researchers from the University of Texas did some brain scans of men, only to observe that the pleasure-reward sites in their brains lit up when they viewed pictures of women's booties.

Butts are the new boobs! Butts are the sexy of all time.

Several years ago, I started doing magazine shoots. It was around that time that my own butt began to attract a lot of attention. I humbly admit that my bottom is tight and perky. If I walked backward into a room, people would check it out perhaps with a smirk. My booty is the one part of my body that is a staple of looking pretty good. Not a bad thing, really. Hair has its good days and bad days. And depending on what I eat, my tummy is either presentable or not. But my butt is always in good shape no matter how the rest of me looks or feels, and the rest of my body is my booty's accessory. Women want to know my secrets for achieving this level of definition, tone and sculpted booty. I'm unveiling my secrets here for that tight booty!

What you may not realize is that the butt is one of the easiest body parts to transform. It is a simple equation to master: the right diet + some kick-ass (excuse the pun) workouts = a sexy rear view that stands out loud and proud in every outfit. No padded jeans or underwear needed for a booty-licious body!

In case you're wondering how this book came about, let me give you a quick rundown. For the past ten years, I've built a career in the fitness industry that has involved owning a gym, training moms, young and old athletes, grandmothers, celebrities, Olympians, and others. I give nutrition seminars all over the world, and I compete in fitness and Olympic weightlifting competitions. Along the way, I was the first woman to be a full-time member of a NASCAR pit crew in the highest level Cup series, changing superheavy tires on race cars as fast as I could.

After I hung up my NASCAR firesuit and put away my tire-changing air wrench, I devoted my life to inspiring people to get in shape and realize the bodies of their dreams.

But let me say this: My butt and my body—and indeed my life—wasn't always in such great shape. The fundamental problem I had was that I did not believe in myself. I struggled with self-doubt as a kid. I was angry and unhappy, and I didn't feel worthy of love. I had no self-worth, and all I could see were obstacles in from of me. I abused my body with alcohol, drugs, and cigarettes.

I was not always the Christmas Abbott you see today.

Then, through some amazing experiences, I stopped playing small and insignificant. I grew in confidence and changed not just my body but my whole life in a positive way.

Let me share my story. I hope it will inspire you to create the body and the fulfillment you want in your own life.

WHO AM I?

I was a Christmas baby, born December 20.

Bet you guessed that one. While pregnant with me, my mom had to stay in bed for several months in order to avert a miscarriage. Even in the womb, I guess I was damn determined to be a part of this world, and so I punched right out, much to the delight of my mom. In gratitude, she named me Christmas Joye. I was teased and made fun of a lot because of that name, so I kept to myself a lot and was a quiet but happy little girl.

I was raised mostly in Lynchburg, Virginia, the middle child in a family with three kids. We lived in a range of homes, mostly lower income, but moved around quite often, always roaming with my father's job. My brother slept in a hallway of our house; my sister and I shared a bed at one point, but at least we had a bedroom. I lived a nomadic lifestyle from the get-go, surrounded by bikers and hippies.

Since childhood, I've always been a contradiction. I loved to wear dresses, but I also loved to climb trees. At age nine, I wanted to play baseball rather than girls' softball—not to make a gender-related statement, but because a baseball fit better in my small hand. The league I tried to join originally told me I couldn't play. Only after my mother threatened to tell the media about the issue did they let me on the team as the only girl. I was also a cheerleader at the same time. But after that, my athletic career ended, and by the time I was a teenager, I was no longer involved in sports.

Growing up, I was never pushed to do much, although I was raised in a loving household. I didn't think anyone had any big dreams for me; I certainly had none for myself. I just felt that I wouldn't be something or do anything important or even impressive. As a result, I couldn't do anything without making a mess of it. So I didn't play sports, I didn't study, I didn't do much of anything productive. I couldn't find one thing that I excelled at or that gave me confidence. I turned into a troubled child and felt destined to be complacent at life. I became a wild child.

At age 13, I was in a horrific car accident. I got out alive with only a scar on my hand, while my sister, Kole, landed in a coma and almost died. The doctors said she wouldn't last through the night. But she did. Then they said she wouldn't wake up. But she did. Then they claimed she would never walk again. But she did.

Thank God, Kole healed—a testimony to the toughness for which the women in my family are known. Still, I was angry about what happened to my sister, and I felt guilty. I had to undergo therapy. It helped somewhat, but there were residual emotional scars.

As a teenager, I started smoking and drinking. I partied as much as possible at every opportunity—which was often. Some people I was hanging out with were experimenting with some heavy-duty drugs, and I went right along with them. Little by little, I was digging myself deeper into a hole of despair.

I was in a downward spiral, depressed and on a one-way track to addiction.

I tried the college scene for about a year, subsisting on ramen noodles for food, but the tuition was too expensive to pay up front. I didn't have the funds to go full time without a loan, and I didn't want any debt.

By then my mother had left for Iraq, working as a civilian, and convinced me to apply for a job there too. I was hired. At age 22, I followed her to Baghdad and took a job in the city's International Zone, once home to Saddam Hussein's ministries and palaces. I was still smoking, drinking, and grossly out of shape, living on the fringe of a very dangerous lifestyle.

I was employed as a laundry attendant to support the US military. Soldiers would bring me their laundry. I'd sort it, ticket it, and issue it back to them when clean. That's what I did 12 hours a day, every day, in a desert war zone.

It was a scary time, with the sound of mortar fire and powerful explosions reverberating all around me constantly, as if heaven and earth had collided. Plumes of smoke would darken the sky, dust swirled into our eyes, and we'd all run for cover. Each time, my heart felt like it had leaped out of my chest.

I realized that if or when something happened, there were two possibilities. The military would carry me out with them, or they would leave me there. The likelihood of someone carrying me into safety in that environment was slim to none. I'd be abandoned there, because I'd be too weak to escape on my own.

The possibility of death was ever-present. It was in the midst of a mortar attack that I realized where I was in my life—not geographically, but rather lifestyle-wise. For too long, I had recklessly taken risks with my health, and I knew if I wasn't careful they'd be the cause of my demise. In short, I was killing myself with my own bad habits. In one of those "life's too short" epiphanies, it hit me that I have choices. I thought: *Am I better than this? I don't have to live this way, and I don't want to die.*

I decided to change my habits and the way I was living. I adjusted my diet by cutting out alcohol and fried, greasy junk, and I started eating healthier food. I stopped smoking, cold turkey. This was the hardest thing I had ever done in my life, but it made me realize that if I put my mind to something positive, I could feel good and reap the rewards of accomplishment.

A few months after quitting smoking, I tried to run a mile, but my cigarette-singed lungs held me back. Running hurt and I hated it. I wanted to quit, but a friend wouldn't let me. "It's only a mile!" he urged. I pressed on, with more of a speed walk than a run. It took me a week to recover from that mile. Running was definitely not for me.

Many months later, a coworker convinced me to try some light gym workouts with him. At first I thought this was beyond my abilities—I was pretty much a weakling—but I gave it a try. I started out lightly. I felt awkward and embarrassed at first. Girls working out in this desert environment were rare. I fumbled around on the machines. My friend encouraged me to stick with it, and I found that my body responded with surprising speed. Results! For the first time in my life, I saw positive changes in my body. I really got into it, and eventually started to enjoy the workouts. I learned more about weight training and figured out how to push my body. I made a commitment to myself when I started to discover fitness.

I then began training with a group of Special Forces guys who literally wanted to break me. Picture this: little tiny me, at five feet, three inches, so underweight at 95 to 100 pounds that I looked anorexic. You could see the bones in my chest as clearly as on a skeleton. There I was, working out with these big husky macho soldiers! They'd put me through horrific workouts, standing over me to make sure I did every part of the workout and forcing me to finish. What would take them 15 minutes took me 30 to 45 minutes. Barely able to keep up, I was embarrassed and always the last to finish.

After a few of those grueling workouts, those guys were convinced that I'd stop showing up. But I returned every day, knowing they were waiting for me with a hell workout.

My tenacity and determination to hang in there earned their respect. But really, I learned a valuable lesson from them: *Do not give up, no matter what.* That lesson stuck with me and would become the foundation for success in my life.

Through this rigorous weight training and decent nutrition, I also discovered that I could transform myself into a person of great strength—outside and inside—by getting out of my comfort zone and taking on new challenges. I was still afraid to take risks, but I no longer allowed that fear to deter me from doing so, and I wasn't afraid to fail.

One day, I met a marine who showed me a video of some girls doing pull-ups, squats, and power cleans. They were totally defined, sculpted, and strong. They had tight butts and flat bellies. I couldn't believe my eyes. I wanted a body like theirs. I wanted a butt like theirs. I wanted to push myself like they did. They were CrossFit athletes. I wanted to be one of them.

And eventually, I was—and more.

THE CROSSFIT CHALLENGE

I'm a quirky person who likes to play, and CrossFit looked to me like an adult playground. There were balls to throw, sleds to pull, sandbags to carry, wooden boxes to jump on, and of course, barbells, dumbbells, kettlebells, and all sorts of fun stuff to play with. A strength and conditioning program favored by police, military personnel, and elite athletes, CrossFit challenges your body at many different levels, and you can constantly change your workouts, even on a daily basis. I started my CrossFit athletic journey in 2006 and have loved every painful minute since.

CrossFit also awakened me to the importance of good nutrition—quality proteins, carbohydrates, and fats—for energy, esthetics, and performance. I changed the way I had been eating—no more junk food, haphazard eating, and reckless nutritional choices. In order to compete successfully at the level I desired, I began to look at food as muscle fuel—something that could help me change my body composition toward more muscle and less fat, plus give me the energy to train all-out. I tightened up on my nutrition and got super-serious about it. This knowledge and practice eventually led to the nutrition plans you'll read about in this book.

I got so immersed in the CrossFit subculture that I eventually opened my own gym—called CrossFit Invoke—in Raleigh in 2010. I even decided to enter the CrossFit Games. At these events, individual competitors and teams undergo a wide variety of athletic events that include challenges such as Olympic lifts, gymnastics, running, powerlifting, rowing, rope climbs, swimming, kettlebell swings, obstacle courses, and a lot more.

In 2010, I competed in the CrossFit Sectionals and Regionals. My goals were simple: I wanted to finish every workout, and I wanted to finish in the top 50 percent. Out of sixty-three female contestants in the regionals, I placed fifth at Sectionals and twentieth at Regionals, and was proud of it.

I have competed in the CrossFit Games Open every year since then, returning to Regionals four times, the Games twice, and in countless smaller CrossFit competitions. I always enjoy my experience and have a great time with the CrossFit community. I won so many events that I soon became nationally ranked in both CrossFit events and Olympic Weightlifting, where I compete at the 53-kilo level. You wouldn't believe it if you saw me, but I can deadlift 270 pounds. CrossFit training made me that strong.

Olympic weightlifting competition is grueling and demands tons of strength and technique. It involves performing movements called the snatch and the clean and jerk. With the snatch, you hoist a barbell off the floor in one continuous motion over your head. Next, you pull your whole body under it so that you're standing with your elbows locked in extension with the weight overhead, then stand to finish the lift.

The clean and jerk are two movements performed in one session. With the clean, you pull the weighted barbell to your shoulders. Immediately afterward you do the jerk, by hoisting the same weight overhead and finishing in a standing position with the weight overhead.

It's all very intense, but this style of training has given me results I wouldn't see through any other workout program—and it was a life-changer for me. CrossFit made me an athlete.

I still compete today, and it has become a part of my life. I love competing, the preparation it takes and the lifestyle. I can't imagine doing anything else. Winning is wonderful, but the greatest reward is inspiring others to go for a goal and realize their dreams.

NASCAR COMES CALLING

In 2012, a friend I'd met through CrossFit called and asked if I wanted to be recruited for something called NASCAR Day. Sure, why not? Another new experience. Right up my alley.

Off I went, wearing a cute little workout outfit ready to drive a car. Whoops! To my surprise, I ended up doing pit crew and didn't drive any of the cars. I wouldn't have gone had I known that.

For one thing, I certainly wasn't interested in changing tires—that is, until I held the air gun and hit lug nuts for the first time. I was instantly hooked. Similar to CrossFit events, we had a competition to see how fast we could jack the car, hang a tire, and hit lug nuts. I was able to jack the car but not very well. Give me a break—it weighs more than 4,000 pounds! I was very accurate with hanging the tire, though, and when it came to hitting lug nuts, that was when I had the most fun. I nailed it. I was the only girl there and beat all the guys with my hand speed of 1.7 seconds per five lug nuts. The hand speed for NASCAR Cup is 1.2 seconds. So even on my first day, I was hitting lug nuts almost as fast as professional pit crewers. Everyone saw me do all this, but they were still shocked. They couldn't believe this kind of performance came from a girl who stood only five feet three and weighed 118 pounds.

Pit crews are vital in every race. They're the often-unsung behind-the-scenes people who play a pivotal part in a race car driver's success. What the driver can't make up on the racetrack, time-wise, that pit crew has to make up in the pits. A smooth pit stop is a well-choreographed athletic feat. Six men (before I came along) are asked to change four tires, add gasoline, and sometimes make a spring adjustment in under 15 seconds. One loose lug nut can mean catastrophe.

Pit crew members are sought out for their body type, agility, accuracy, and strength. Everyone on a pit crew is either a former pro athlete or a collegiate athlete, all incredibly skilled. I was none of the above.

Pit crewing originally wasn't meant to be a woman's job, but I'm no ordinary woman. I crave new challenges. I'm someone who pushes the envelope at every turn and still, a real study in contrast, as I mentioned. I love lipstick, stiletto heels—and tattoos. I have a gun tattooed on my hip to remind me of my days in Iraq and how they got me on the straight-and-narrow fitness path. I'm as girlie as they get with dresses and glam, but I'm also as ferocious as they come, with a tenacity to conquer my goal and win.

Not long afterward, I got a call from Turner Motorsport. Was I interested in pit crewing for real? With a laugh, I said that the tryout was fun, but I'd had no idea it was such a brute-force job. In absolute amazement of what came out of my mouth next, I admitted that I loved changing tires.

However, I had a full plate at the time. I was managing my CrossFit gym, coaching most of the classes, teaching bodyweight boot camps, doing fitness seminars almost every weekend, and training for CrossFit competitions. I was already a fitness celebrity and model with a lot going on. Thanks, but no thanks.

But I kept thinking about it. I started researching pit crew development and anything else I could find out about this fascinating new endeavor. I became obsessed with learning more. I hadn't found something that fascinated me this much since I discovered CrossFit. All I could think about was pit crewing

It would be tough, for sure. CrossFit had taken me to a higher level of achievement. NASCAR could take me beyond. The idea gnawed at me. I reached the moment of, "Damn, I'll do it."

Eventually, I joined the Michael Waltrip Racing Team and held the distinction of being the first and only female full-time member of a NASCAR pit crew at the Cup level, the sport's highest level of professional competition. All week, I'd be out at practice for training drills to build technique and muscle memory. We'd rehearse pit stops so that on race day we'd be as quick, strong, and focused as possible. We'd look at videotapes of our previous performance. Every pit stop is videotaped so the crews can later study time and motion. It was highly technical work, with no room for even the tiniest mistake, and I loved every minute of it.

At the racetrack, I stood poised on the pit wall, ready with my weight forward on my toes, waiting for just the right split second to spring across the lane as the car pulled into the pit box. When it decelerated toward me, I dove off the wall with a long right-legged stride to cover as much ground as fast as possible to get to the far side of the car.

I eyed the front right tire and anticipated the very instant at which the car would stop. That way, I could thrust myself onto the ground in the exact position to hit the first lug nut the moment the car stopped. With my hands moving as fast and as accurately as humanly possible, I punched my air gun over every lug nut on the front tires, ripped them off, and pounded five new lug nuts onto the new tire with absolute consistence and precision. All in around 14 seconds flat. In a sport where a split second can make all the difference, the agility and athleticism of the pit crew often decides who wins and who loses.

Pit crewing is a dangerous job, too. You're a sitting duck in that pit box. You can be struck by another driver or even your own driver. It's an all-out active game of chicken, but no one backs down or gets out of the way.

I lived and breathed NASCAR. If you came to my house, you'd see a garage full of training equipment and a kitchen counter strewn with lug nuts, worn gloves, duct tape to keep my knee pads on, and oil everywhere. I kept my first lug nut from my debut race at the Daytona 500. The lug nut is pink, and it's a souvenir I treasure.

Being a NASCAR pit crew member meant everything to me, but mostly I felt I was a role model. I was showing young women everywhere that anything is possible, and that they have the opportunity to make better decisions for themselves every day of their lives. There's plenty of room for women in this sport.

Most people carry the negative and limiting voices of childhood around with them all their lives. I'm thankful that I did not. My feelings of inadequacy made me determined to try new things, step out on unfamiliar paths, and not give up on myself. Everything I was told I couldn't do, I've done. My success all came down to taking action for myself.

That's what I'd like you to do—take action. With this book, I'm going to challenge those of you who have put off your own fitness and health for too long. If I can go from a nonathletic, out-of-shape girl—what I call a misfit—to MissFit woman, you can too. I'm here to help you.

I love to show that as a woman, you can own your body and have a complete say in how it looks. If you want that, it's yours to take, but rewards this great do not come without effort. If you want to sit on your couch and *think* about crunches, pick up another book and be happy with your body as it is now. Otherwise, with me, you'll venture into a fun, short, intense, and creative program that gets you in amazing shape fast!

You have the power to change your life and your body for the better every day you wake up. It's a decision you have to work at every day: to take control of your body, and to care for yourself so you can move through the world with real confidence. The power to do that is yours to take, not anyone else's.

You don't have to have any previous fitness experience or sports experience to do my program. I certainly didn't. You simply have to be willing to try and give it what you have! Along the way, start imagining how sexy you're going to look in those booty-fitting jeans, bikini, and short shorts—and how sexy and confident you'll feel looking in your own mirror.

Are you ready? Then follow me.

THE BADASS BODY DIET

PART 1

GET YOUR REAR IN GEAR

Getting a Badass Body

BE THRILLED THAT YOU picked up this book, because I'm going to show you how to get a tight ass and an overall lean, sexy body—without all the BS of dumb DIE-ts (yes, that's how I spell it), miracle fixes, and fluffy exercises. Nope—none of that. I'm going to cut through all that crap and get you into the shape of your life—and show you the amazing lifestyle change that will allow you to stay there.

I developed this program in response to my own struggle with food and my desire to be able to eat whatever I wanted. Anyone who knows me will tell you I have an appetite. I love to eat, so I needed a plan that would let me enjoy food and ultimately change my body to look and feel the way I wanted it to. That is, more muscle and less body fat. Could this be done without severely restricting food? I wasn't sure.

I went to work, researching various approaches to dieting. Most of the diets I read about were ridiculous: too extreme, restrictive, super complicated, and mostly fads. Still, I persevered. I ended up taking the best parts of certain diets and "Frankensteining" them into the best combo for me. I admit there was a lot of trial and error, but the result was a way of eating that was lower in carbohydrates, higher in fat, high in protein—and with some room for "controlled cheating," which would give me a dose of reality in my eating habits. From everything I researched, these elements were key to successful weight loss if you wanted it and muscle gain—which is what I wanted. Along the way, I identified "booty foods" that could actually help reduce fat from the lower body. I included those foods in my program too.

Of course, food wouldn't the only way toward a great booty and body. Exercise had to be an influencing component, though not the biggest one. Our bodies are more than just food-processing machines. They're designed to play, move, and discover life. When you deny yourself the joy and power of movement, you plunge yourself into a vicious cycle of lack of motivation and binge eating.

Here's another thing: I'm advocating a nondiet—and more of a change in the way you eat and see food, specifically the big three "macronutrients," protein, fat, and carbohydrates. The Badass Body Diet is something you can do daily and live with forever—and with a few modifications and adjustments in portion size, your guy can do it with you.

Diets always fail, but understanding your food and what it can do for you is key to making permanent and positive changes. With this book, you now have the knowledge to see food differently and make better, smarter choices.

Ultimately, the exercises I included in my plan were strength-based and designed to activate a lot of muscle groups at once, particularly those in the thighs and buttocks. The workouts are short but intense, meant to not only firm up muscles but provide aerobic conditioning while taking into consideration how important your time is. Pairing my food plan with exercise, even only three times a week, will rocket your body into a transformation that you won't believe.

I put my diet and exercise program to the test, using a single guinea pig: myself. My body started to change. I was getting leaner, but stronger and defined to precision. I was able to stay at the top of my weight class in Olympic Weightlifting. My rear end had gotten tight and free of cellulite.

My CrossFit clients took notice. They were curious about exactly what I was doing, and they wanted the same results.

Because their bodies were different from mine, I knew the program would need to adapt a little, so I eventually tweaked it to fit everyone and every lifestyle: the woman who wants a more aesthetic shape, the woman who has never done anything athletic or healthy in her life, the athlete who wants to perform better, and the seeker of more energy and a happier state of being. I wanted to include everyone and make it comprehensive enough for anyone.

The Badass Body Diet was born.

HOW IT WORKS: BADASS NUTRITION

How many times have you asked, "Does my butt look big in this?" Whether you're dragging your boyfriend, hubby, or best friend through hell by trying on every outfit in your closet until you get a satisfactory answer, the question is always loaded, and you know your butt looks as big as Jupiter if you're even asking the question.

To improve your rear reflection and the rest of you, you'll follow my Badass nutrition plan. It focuses on clean, high-protein eating—with a twist: it's a bit higher in fat than most diets you've probably been on. Once upon a time, fat was the "F" word—everyone thought it was very bad for your waistline and everywhere else. Sounds like a crazy idea, but many more recent studies have shown that dietary fat isn't the bad guy. Half the composition of your cell membranes is fat, so it's essential for healthy functioning. Fat is also key for absorbing fat-soluble vitamins like vitamin A, which encourages protein turnover and, indirectly, muscle growth.

Eating fat doesn't mean you'll get fat. In fact, consuming the right amount of certain fats can help you shed body fat, develop muscle, defend your joints, protect your heart, and make food taste better. So hello, dietary fat, good-bye, body fat!

You won't feel hungry on my program, either, because you'll be eating enough protein and higher-fat foods. Ultimately, you'll feel satisfied instead of deprived. You'll see and feel the pounds fall off—from your stomach first, since this is where fat from carbs is typically stored, and then from your booty, thighs, and entire lower body.

Be prepared to go pretty low on certain carbs. You've got to. When you take in too many carbs, your blood sugar elevates, and then the hormone insulin kicks in to bring it back down. In doing so, it takes the calories you've consumed and stores them as fat. And this fat is hard to get rid of, wants to stay put, and creates cellulite. If you ever find you're getting fat, you haven't adjusted your carbs properly

I won't deny it: The low-carb approach works. A ton of research tells us that curtailing carbs causes dramatic drops in body fat. When you skimp on certain carbs and lower their overall intake, your body produces less glucose and stops creating fatty tissue. Your body turns to existing fat reserves to burn energy, so you lose weight.

I do make distinctions among carbs, though. I discourage carbs such pasta, cereal, bread, crackers, desserts, and processed foods, especially those with commercial brand labels with long lists of crazy ingredients, additives, and chemicals. If it has such a label, stay away! But don't panic: I have a ton of great alternatives for these if they are a part of your life that you can't let go of.

My dietary plan also includes some specific foods that can literally spot-reduce your butt. Yep, there are foods that will do this, and they're the centerpiece of my diet. I call them "booty foods." Think: meat and other animal proteins, fruits, vegetables, and yes, fats. Don't run yet; let me explain! With the right protein, fat, and carb choices, you'll burn up fat that is already stored on various parts of your body and produce rapid results to give you the motivation to create your ideal body. Of course, you get to eat many more foods than just my booty foods, because the Badass plan offers a lot of variety.

You'll enjoy breakfast, lunch, dinner, and snacks. Each meal is made up of proteins, carbohydrates, and fats designed to help you achieve the perfect posterior and shape—and a goddess-like bod in and out of clothes.

Fair warning: I've always challenged rules, so why have diet rules? I'm going to break a bunch of them. Don't freak out. This plan works, and I've seen it transform the booties and bodies of everyone I've worked with. Go at it with courage and boldness. After all, as they say, tame women rarely make history.

I'M A BADASS!

First comes love, then comes marriage. But between the two, a lot of women get to the altar with considerably more than what they should weigh. My client Cathy is a good example. She was gearing up for her wedding, six months away—and that was incentive enough for her to starting making changes.

Cathy started one of my plans at around 30 percent body fat. She's five feet five inches tall, with a curvy, hourglass figure. Naturally, she wanted to trim down as much as possible to look the best ever in her wedding gown.

Her usual diet wasn't very nutritious, with hardly any veggies or fruit, so we changed all that. Cathy started buying more produce and got rid of all the junk food in her house. I introduced her to high-protein eating and showed her how to enjoy some yummy fats like peanut butter and sour cream. She discovered that by eating six meals a day, she never felt deprived. Cathy coupled Badass nutrition with my workout, exercising just three times a week.

By the end of the first month, Cathy had dropped four whole dress sizes and trimmed her booty considerably, completing her six-month goal in only 30 days. After the wedding, she continued to practice Badass habits, firmed up even more, and stayed in superior shape.

HOW IT WORKS: BADASS WORKOUTS

Right now, you might not like the idea of exercising. I hear you. I used to hate to exercise. But I gave it a whirl and kept at it. Once I saw positive changes in my body, I felt like I was doing something good for myself that only I could do and couldn't be bought. I always feel like a million bucks after working out. I know I've done something positive for myself, and this builds my confidence. Exercise also biochemically changes your system. It boosts feel-good chemicals like serotonin and endorphins, and it increases muscle-toning chemicals such as growth hormone and testosterone. Not to mention that exercise also increases your sex drive.

Getting a firm, sexy ass and body must involve the right kinds of exercises and work-outs, and you'll find them here. Just as you'll eat foods to spot-reduce your butt, you'll do exercises that will spot-firm it. Diet and exercise—it's like a combo punch. No body part escapes my exercise program, however, because it's not a good idea to work only your butt. You need to work off fat from everywhere to create the whole beautiful body package. My workouts tax your entire body, making it tough for any muscle part to goof off—which increases the effects of the workout. They're fast-paced, too, with constant motion that aerobically elevates your heart rate and burns calories like crazy.

Sometimes women don't want to do weight training because they're afraid they'll bulk up. You don't have to worry about that, because for men, the muscular bodybuilder physique comes from male hormones as much as it does from lifting weights. We just don't have the same hormonal makeup. The workouts here will firm, tone, and strengthen your body without bulking it up.

You don't have to spend hours exercising, either. My exercises are easy to follow and accompanied by step-by-step pictures and instructions. None of my workouts lasts longer than 20 minutes, and I offer variety and levels of ability for everyone, from the absolute Badass beginner to the elite Badass babe.

If you follow my workouts closely, you'll get a rock-solid sexy body that sizzles in skinny jeans, bikinis, and other clothes, and turns heads and literally stops traffic. And that's the truth.

WHAT'S IT GONNA TAKE?

Maybe you're a little reluctant or timid right now, because you've tried so many programs that have failed you. You're sick of the word *diet*. You're tired of exercises being pushed at you. Okay, fine. I get that too. But let's look at this another way.

Think of the first time you had sex. It was awkward, a real fumble fest. You didn't really know what was exactly going on. You weren't even sure you liked it. But you tried it again and again. After more weird tries, you started to like it. Soon you loved it.

Well, it's just like that with the Badass plan. You start it. You fumble a bit. You keep at it. You see amazing results, and then you love it. It becomes a part of your life.

I want to help you get there by sharing with you what I call the three Cs of success: clarity, confidence, and consistency.

CLARITY

By clarity, I mean being honest with yourself about where you are, where you want to be, and what you really want out of life. I advise my clients to keep a journal in which they clearly describe how they want to look and the goals for getting there. To start the process, I urge them to use visualization, a relatively old concept in the field of sport psychology used for performance enhancement. Before you start my plan, visualize your healthy ideal and describe it in your journal. Create the picture, feel it, and then hold it intently in your mind. See yourself already at your ideal. According to research, the mind controls the body by directing and moving it toward the visualized image. Another way to put it is, what you believe, you conceive.

Also, write down the concrete goals you can take to actualize that vision. How much weight loss is your ultimate goal? Ten pounds? Twenty-five? Fifty? Or perhaps enough to finally squeeze back into those jeans that have become too tight in recent months? Maybe it's not so much about losing weight but rather getting that smoking-hot body shaped up. Feel free to make your goals as challenging as you like. This is, after all, your life.

Next, list what you're willing to sacrifice to achieve your goals. Every accomplishment worth anything didn't come without sacrifice. Understanding what you want and what it takes to get it is the important part. You're stronger than you think—you just have to be willing to try.

During my own fitness makeover, it was obvious to me that I'd have to give up dearly beloved long-term habits such as drinking, smoking, and eating junk food full of fats and sugar. Be brutally honest about the bad habits you'll give up. Will you stop eating fast food or nightly desserts? Will you give up daily cocktails? How about those daily sodas you've been knocking down? Will you stop being sedentary? Will you refrain from medicating yourself with food when you feel stressed out? Your bad habits are standing in your way. Don't let this insignificant bad habit prevent you from the body you know you can have. Be your own boss, kick those bad habits to the curb, and replace them with good habits. That's the Badass way.

Be clear, too, about your priorities. Women are always concerned about taking care of others first. This isn't a bad thing, but it can be problematic when you don't value your well-being enough to put it at the top of your priority list. How can you take care of others properly unless you take care of yourself first? Priorities change depending on the situation; values do not. At first, eating well and working out will be priorities and require active vigilance; then, as you see positive changes in your body, those priorities shift into values and a way of life.

CONFIDENCE

Confidence is the belief that you'll be successful in a given situation, but it's not something we necessarily come by naturally, and it ebbs and flows. Few of us escape feelings of fear and self-doubt as we go about our lives.

I know, because I used to have zero confidence. I rebelled because I was scared of failure and afraid of what people thought. I figured if I didn't try or care, then I'd never fail. However, I was just letting myself down. It wasn't until I decided that I deserved more that I was able to turn my life around. Honestly, it was a struggle at times. Big changes always are. But I knew I wanted a better life, able to reach my eighties and still take care of myself without assistance. I didn't do it just for the body—I did it for long-term quality of life.

I started with baby steps, nothing huge or life-altering. Every tiny step I took in the right direction brought better outcomes, plus the confidence that comes with those results. You can build confidence in the same way.

If you've habitually failed at diets, for example, you probably struggle with self-confidence. That's when you need to take little steps yourself. One way to do this is what I call "layering changes." For example, start with just a breakfast change in which you eat a healthy morning meal. Once you've nailed your breakfast, move to lunch changes, then dinner changes. Layering looks like this:

Week 1: Eat a nutritious breakfast all week.
Week 2: Eat a nutritious breakfast and lunch all week.
Week 3: Eat a nutritious breakfast, lunch, and dinner all week.

One change at a time, one meal at a time—that's layering. It gives you small wins, and your confidence grows.

At times, you'll hear voices of self-doubt in your mind, telling you that you can't do something, that you'll fail, or that you're not good enough. These voices undermine your confidence. I still struggle with these disempowering voices, but I've learned how to shut them up. Every time I hear one, I just tell myself aloud, "I'm worth it" or "I deserve better" or "I'll triumph over this." And my favorite: "You're the baddest bitch here—show them you are!"

You can choose your thoughts and therefore control your emotions. You have the natural ability to cancel any thought that makes you feel bad or depressed. When negative mind chatter starts sounding off, replace it with a more empowering voice, such as "I can do this," "I'm strong today," "I'm grateful for what I have," or "I'm in control of my body and my life." Not only will you increase your confidence and success dramatically, but eventually, those negative voices will get quieter and quieter as they recognize they have little influence on you.

As you and I go through my program together, I realize you might not initially have the confidence that you can change your body and your life. That's okay! You don't have to believe it now to start it. Eventually, though, that belief will come, when you see the results and feel the difference in your strength, energy, and overall well-being. You'll become a believer in your own power to be better than you've ever been. And others will notice!

CONSISTENCY

Consistency means staying the course—no yo-yoing between virtuous salads and "screw-it" cheesecakes in any given week, no exercising one or two days a week, then couch-slouching the rest. The secret behind maintaining consistency is to take a day-by-day approach. If you want to improve, concentrate on what you have to do *today* only. Each "today" adds up—to a week, a month, two months, six months, a lifetime.

What if you backslide? Don't beat yourself up over it. Just start anew at the next meal or the next workout. My old pit crew coach used to tell me, "We all fail, but you need to fail quickly and move on."

What matters is how you respond to failure. Are you going to dwell on it and let it control you? Or are you going to accept that you're human, apply the lesson, and move forward? Get back on the program immediately, be patient with yourself, and stay in charge of your own life.

Approaching the program this way will give you better results, faster. Fitness success is a daily habit, not a once-in-a-while, when-you-have-time sort of thing.

OKAY . . . NOW FOR THE PERKS

When I'm done with you, you'll have an amazing body shape—the perfect balance of hourglass curves and defined booty, tummy, and everywhere in between.

You'll love the results: Up to five pounds will blitz off your body in just the first few days, as will inches. Part of this is due to water loss within muscle cells—but that's a positive. Waterlogged cells are partly responsible for that ugly look called cellulite. Getting rid of excess water, aka bloat, along with body fat, minimizes the appearance of cellulite on your hips and thighs. The initial pounds you shed will be due to water loss, but after just a few days, you'll also start to burn fat.

Going forward, there are some other important benefits that you can't see but you'll feel: endurance and strength. Everyday activities on the job, housework, or yard work will be less tiring. You'll sleep better at night. Your sex life will improve, and you'll have more energy for all sorts of activities. And don't be surprised if you start walking around with a sexy strut because you love your new look.

My plan isn't just about having a sexy bod and booty; it's also about being empowered. Being in shape gives you a positive mind-set, which in turn boosts confidence and improves self-esteem. Your thinking will be sharper, and you'll be able to focus better, with a degree of mental clarity you haven't experienced in a while. You might not be able to control everything that happens to you, but you can control your level of fitness and how you perceive yourself.

Decide today to make better choices for yourself the same way I did years ago. You earned your opportunity to be here, taking a chance on yourself right now. Take it!

It's never too late to change for the better, either. My mother was in her fifties when she quit smoking, and she'd smoked for thirty years. She just started CrossFitting a couple of years ago too. She's is a true testament how you can start wherever you are, and make positive changes that last.

Once you make the right choices, you'll change your life too. And you can do it through good food, fun exercises, and a hot booty to show for all of your hard work. Give yourself a chance to amaze yourself!

Now I'd like to give you a short course on that booty of yours—and how we're going to pry off the resistant pudge.

CHAPTER 2

The Skinny on Your Butt

MEET YOUR BUTT.

Maybe you haven't seen it in a while, what with it being behind you all the time. Or maybe you've been camouflaging it with that really long black dress. I declare those days over. You're about to get the best, sexiest booty in town. And you should flaunt it!

But first you've got to understand a little physiology about that sweet ass of yours—in order to understand how to get it in shape.

THE GLUTES—THREE MUSCLES IN ONE

Your butt is actually composed of three muscles: the gluteus maximus, gluteus medius, and gluteus minimus (collectively known as the "glutes"). I consider them perhaps the coolest muscles of the body, and collectively the biggest trio of muscles you have. They do a lot of work. They help you climb up stairs, walk and run, jump, pivot, play sports, get on and off the toilet, and, ahem, assist in lovemaking.

But our modern and inactive lifestyles—including long commutes, desk jobs, and TV watching—mean our glutes aren't getting the exercise they require. This idleness is triggering problems, especially in the back. If your glutes aren't strong, you'll be susceptible to back pain. And of course, a droopy butt will prevail!

Love 'em or hate 'em, remember this: glutes are muscles. And like all muscles, they can be toned up, especially with the exercises in this book.

A BIG BUTT IS NOT HEALTHY

By "not healthy," I'm talking about flabby, out-of-shape butts, not tight, firm, muscled butts that might be a little big. A lot of fat on the hips is unhealthy. Let me explain.

We carry fat on different parts of our bodies—a fat distribution technically known as a "fat pattern." Some people have a type of fat pattern called *upper body obesity* or *central obesity*. Those are the folks with big bellies. They're at a higher risk for scary illnesses such as diabetes, heart disease, and certain cancers.

The other type of fat pattern is termed *lower body obesity*. This means that you carry most of your fat on your hips, buttocks, and thighs.

Used to be, medical science geeks said that it was okay—even healthy—if you carried more body fat on your lower body. In fact, this type of fat patterning was once thought to protect against illness, particularly diabetes and heart disease.

Oh, how science changes its mind.

New research indicates that pear-shaped bodies are not healthier than apple-shaped physiques. In 2013, scientists at UC Davis Health System published a fascinating study in *The Journal of Clinical Endocrinology and Metabolism*. Their study revealed that it could be dangerous to your health to carry a lot of fat on the lower body. That's because fat in the buttocks area churns out high levels of *chemerin* and not enough *omentin-1*. These proteins, when out of balance, can lead to chronic inflammation and prediabetes. The people in the study who had a lot of chemerin, for example, also had high blood pressure, elevated levels of C-reactive protein (a sign of inflammation), high triglycerides, problems processing insulin, and low levels of HDL cholesterol (the good kind). Similarly, the subjects with low omentin-1 had high triglycerides and blood sugar and low levels of HDL cholesterol. So basically, booty fat appears to mess up factors that protect us from dangerous diseases.

Where lower body fat is concerned, another health problem is osteoarthritis, a crippling joint disease that affects millions of people. Any extra pounds you carry around on your hips and buttocks exerts wear and tear on your joints—a burden that potentially leads to osteoarthritis. Osteoarthritis doesn't get better, either; it just gets worse as you get older.

All of this is bad news for your heart, bones, and overall health unless you do something about it, like getting a tight butt. Not only will you make healthier food choices but you'll change the level of health and cut the threat of major diseases. A tighter butt might just be saving your life!

BOLLOCKS! BOOTY FAT IS RESISTANT FAT

From a cosmetic standpoint, the frustrating thing about fat around the hips and buttocks is that it's stubborn and clingy, like an old boyfriend you can't shake. But there's a good reason for this clingy fat—the greatest being the support of new life during lactation. When a woman is breast-feeding, the body readily releases lower body fat cells in order to support the energy needs of the nursing baby. Otherwise, fat stored below the waist doesn't surrender easily—but from now on, neither do you!

Understand that fat cell size is regulated by hormone-binding structures on the surface of fat cells called alpha and beta receptors. Receptors attach to hormones and are stimulated in the process. For example, when the beta receptor is stimulated, cells increase their production of lipase, an enzyme that breaks down fat inside the cells. When the alpha receptor is stimulated, however, fat burning is blocked. Fat remains inside, and makes the fat cell even fatter.

We women have more alpha receptors in our lower bodies; men have more in their bellies and chests. The proportion of alpha receptors to beta receptors on fat cells explains why certain parts of your body lose fat faster than others. Surprise, surprise.

Don't freak out if you think you have more alpha than you think you should. By adopting the Badass plan in this book—especially strength training—you can awaken beta receptors, step up the rate at which they burn fat, and deactivate your alpha receptors, making you the alpha woman you were meant to be.

UGH! BOOTY FAT CELLS MULTIPLY

You have about 20 to 30 billion fat cells in your body. Some of this fat is "essential fat." It's the structural constituent of vital body parts such as the brain, nerve tissue, bone marrow, heart, and cell membranes. Women have about 12 to 15 percent essential fat.

You're probably more familiar with the other type of fat: "storage fat." It's what we're always trying to get rid of. Some storage fat pads organs for protection. But most is found just under the skin, and it determines your overall shape.

I'm sure you've heard that when you gain weight, your fat cells expand, and when you lose weight, they shrink. Well, that's true if you're talking about fat cells in and around your belly.

It's a different story for fat cells in your booty. Eat crap like sugar, processed foods, and other calorie-laced junk food, then sit on your ass all day, and guess what? Your butt will start growing extra fat cells! And you've got them for life. Oh no! Extra fat cells is exactly what you don't want.

You can stop population growth in your butt by eating right and exercising a certain way—and drop gobs of this resistant fat in the process.

Hip Advice

1. Stop hating your butt. Resolve to not say things like "Ugh, I hate my butt" or "My butt is too fat." This is a disempowering habit that only ends up hurting your confidence. Repeating negative statements about your body is very damaging, and can undermine your progress. Start to embrace why your body is different, beautiful, and ultimately perfect for you.

2. Bash negative comments with strong positive statements ("My thighs feel so strong when I'm exercising" or "I love how I fill out my pants and dresses now").

3. Post affirming quotes. I keep them in key places in my life to remind me what my goal is and how to stay on track. For example:

—Quote on my fridge: "You are beautiful! Stay the course."
—A few favorite quotes on my bathroom mirror: "Today you can make a change!" "Prove them wrong!"
and "Do today what others won't so you can do tomorrow what others can't."
—Quotes in my car: "Sweat off the fat!" and "I'm doing all this for me!"

4. Get used to how you look and feel when naked. Clean your house in the buff, or wear a bikini while washing your car. Not that bold yet? Then do it in a sexy negligee. The more time you spend naked or nearly naked, the more you'll start loving your body. Check yourself out in the mirror when you get out of the shower. See the changes and feel good about them.

5. Keep at it. My program feeds confidence into you. By the end of the first week, you'll be proud that you make positive changes, such as having a proper breakfast, doing your workouts, and knowing you are on the right track. You'll have the courage to head into week two for even more changes! By the end of the month, you'll be recruiting your friends to experience this new, exciting, and fun way of eating, exercising, and living.

GOOD-BYE, SAG!

There's one thing that will mess up your butt: yo-yo dieting. It can cause your ass to sag, and we don't want droop if we can help it. If you constantly go on and off diets, you'll stretch out and weaken two key protein fibers in your skin: collagen and elastin, both of which make the skin in your butt, and elsewhere, nice and firm. If you keep losing and regaining the same 10 or 20 pounds or more, your butt will sag. It's kind of like washing and stretching out a sweater; eventually the garment wears out. So it is with your butt. Constant dieting worsens the sag, and so does lack of exercise, because those protein fibers endure more stress and consequently break down faster. Your butt goes south.

The Badass plan is one you can embrace for life, because it's flexible and gives you dietary options, depending on where you are in your fitness journey. You can kiss yo-yo dieting good-bye, and keep your ass gorgeous and firm.

BOOHOO! BOOTY FAT AND CELLULITE GO TOGETHER

My friends envy my cellulite-free legs and butt. They're always telling me how lucky I am, but I tell them: "It's not luck, because there's plenty of cellulite in my family tree."

I'm certain the reason I don't have cellulite is that I take care of myself to make sure I stay cellulite free. I believe in the old saying *You are what you eat,* and I know my diet is crucial. I've been a clean eater for years, but with deserved cheat meals. That means no processed foods, no junk food. They take longer to digest and clog up your system; this mess creates cellulite. I don't smoke, either; anything that can impede your blood circulation (such as tobacco) needs to be banned from your lifestyle. And I drink loads of water to flush out my system. Keeping myself hydrated gives me loads of energy too.

Three factors create cellulite: excess body fat, sluggish circulation, and water retention. These factors cause the connective tissue beneath your skin to weaken and collapse. When this happens, fat pushes against your skin, forming dimples. About 90 percent of women have cellulite, especially if we have fat fannies. Sure, every woman who has cellulite hates it. I have yet to meet a woman who wanted more!

If nothing is done about cellulite, skin begins to lose its elasticity and the bulges become more visible. The lymphatic system, which collects and filters damaged cells, bacteria, and viruses, also plays a role. Under normal conditions, it drains fluid from your tissues.

Cellulite, with its trapped fat and weakened tissue, can block this drainage, triggering swelling and thus worsening cellulite.

The "miracle cure" is simple: clean eating, with the right balance of protein, fat, and carbohydrates, along with strength training. There is no other cure—no massage, no cream, no oil, no hope in a jar. If there were one, believe me, I would have found it and told all my clients about it!

Strength training, in particular, develops muscle that helps iron out the appearance of cellulite. Unless you do this form of exercise, your gluteal muscles will stay weak and flaccid. Fat will rest on top of that muscle and produce the lumpy look that we all detest!

Believe me, cellulite does go away. I've seen this happen with the women I train: when they exercise and clean up their diets, it all disappears.

I'M A BADASS

Even though she was fit at 20 percent body fat, Sarah, age 40, was extremely self-conscious about yucky cellulite on her tummy, thighs, and hips and hyperventilated every time beach season rolled around. No matter what she ate or hard she worked out, she couldn't seem to get rid of it.

I started Sarah on one of my plans, emphasizing clean foods only. She did my workout program in conjunction with the plan.

Sarah was motivated and consistent. This paid off in more ways than one.

She dropped about ten more pounds and lowered her body fat percentage to 16. But here's the biggie: By week three, her cellulite was gone. True story.

There's more. She whispered to me that she and her husband were more active in the bedroom than ever before. Her new confidence and sleek body had reignited some hot passion. He can't keep his hands off her!

SEE YA, CELLULITE . . . HELLO, PLEASURE!

Ready to make this all happen? Grab your booty shorts, and let's get prepared for the journey.

CHAPTER 3

My PREP Strategy for Success

I'VE SEEN HUNDREDS OF my clients lose lots of pounds and be successful when they start the program with a strategy that I'm about to share with you.

I call it the PREP Strategy. PREP is an acronym for Photograph (your body), Rate (your weight), Evaluate (your body composition), and Police (your portions). It helps you set benchmarks to evaluate your progress, and see if you're zeroing in on your goals. And it helps you stay the course should your resolve ever start to slip. Use this strategy, and you'll find yourself piling up small successes left and right.

I know you're ready . . . so let's begin.

PHOTOGRAPH YOURSELF

Take several "before" pictures of your whole body and include a "belfie" (butt selfie) the day before you start the program. Do it from different angles—front, side, and back. Ideally, you should wear a two-piece bathing suit if you have one, and take the pictures against a plain background or white wall. If you don't want anyone to see you in a bathing suit, set your camera on a tripod and snap away. Or have a family member or trusted friend click the photos.

I know you probably don't want to do this and would rather wait until you're more "fit," but when you see the changes in your body later, you'll wish you had taken those initial photos. Go ahead and trust me on this. Take the photos and store them away! No one but you has to see these pix.

These pictures are crucial for your success. That's because one of the greatest ways to stay the course is to be able to see your progress—progress that can't be disputed.

When I look back over the last couple of years at my clients who have had the most extreme results, they all took "before" photographs.

RATE YOUR WEIGHT

Most of my clients hate the scales. Just the sight of them makes them break out in a sweat. Those numbers can dictate their moods for the rest of day. Down good; up bad. Down healthy; up, they feel like a slob. I get that, and I'm not a big fan of weighing oneself on scales, either. However, I do think it's important to at least know your weight before you begin. It helps you benchmark your progress going forward. If you decide to weigh yourself regularly, do it just once a week.

But don't be beholden to the numbers on the scale or obsessed with them. Your weight can fluctuate based on fluid retention, constipation, sodium intake, last night's dinner, and other factors that have nothing to do with fat gain.

So before you begin, check your starting weight. Do it in the morning, without clothes. Make a note of that weight, perhaps in a journal.

The following chart gives target weight ranges for women in various age and height groups. Find the ideal range for you. Use that number as the weight-loss goal you'll aim for.

Okay, if you hate the scale like I do, you don't even have to go near it. Just monitor your progress in other ways, such as how your clothes fit or how you look in the mirror in the buff. Both will soon tell a fabulously positive story. Then keep doing the right things and trust that you'll get the right results.

Height	Age (Years)				
	20–29	30–39	40–49	50–59	60–69
4'10"	84–111	92–119	99–127	107–135	115–142
4'11"	87–115	95–123	103–131	111–139	119–147
5'0"	90–119	98–127	106–135	114–143	123–152
5'1"	93–123	101–131	110–140	118–148	127–157
5'2"	96–127	105–136	113–144	122–153	131–163
5'3"	99–131	108–140	117–149	126–158	135–168
5'4"	102–135	112–145	121–154	130–163	140–173
5'5"	106–140	115–149	125–159	134–168	144–179
5'6"	109–144	119–154	129–164	138–174	148–184
5'7"	112–148	122–159	133–169	143–179	153–190
5'8"	116–153	126–163	137–174	147–184	158–196
5'9"	119–157	130–168	141–179	151–190	162–201
5'10"	122–162	134–173	145–184	156–195	167–207
5'11"	126–167	137–178	149–190	160–201	172–213
6'0"	129–171	141–183	153–195	165–207	177–219

Source: Gerontology Research Center, National Institutes of Health

ARE YOU LIVING A BADASS LIFESTYLE?

Take this quiz and learn how you can improve your health and your life as you go through the Badass plan. Read through the multiple choice questions, then circle the letter that best fits your response. Be truthful!

1. Generally, how much shut-eye do you average each night?
   A. Less than six hours
   B. Six to eight hours
   C. More than eight hours

2. When did you get your last medical checkups?

    A. Within the last year

    B. Within last two years

    C. I can't remember

3. How many servings of fruits and vegetables do you eat daily?

    A. Two to four

    B. Hardly any

    C. Five or more

4. How much pure water do you drink each day?

    A. Eight glasses or more

    B. Four to seven glasses

    C. Three or fewer glasses

5. How much exercise do you get each week?

    A. Seven or more hours

    B. Four to six hours

    C. Three or fewer hours

6. How much protein do you eat at meals?

    A. Once a day

    B. At every meal

    C. Several times a week at best

7. How many alcoholic beverages do you drink in a typical week?

    A. None, one, or two

    B. Three to six

    C. Seven or more

8. What is your body fat percentage?

    A. Under 20 percent

    B. Between 20 and 30 percent

    C. Over 30 percent

9. How would you rate your stress level?

A. Moderate

B. Constant

C. I am rarely stressed; I know how to manage it

10. You avoid excess sugar:

A. Most of the time

B. Sometimes

C. Rarely

11. Smoking

A. Trying to quit

B. Never

C. A pack or more daily

12. You have a stable sex partner (or are celibate).

A. Very true

B. Somewhat true

C. I tend to have multiple partners

13. How often do you use illicit drugs?

A. Never

B. Rarely

C. Weekly or more

14. How do you feel about your occupation or what you do for a living?

A. Moderately happy and fulfilled

B. Very happy and fulfilled

C. Unhappy

15. I make time in my schedule for fun, leisure activities, and/or relaxation:

A. Rarely

B. Sometimes

C. Always

1. The best answer is C. Eight to ten hours a night is optimum, though not always practical if you have a busy schedule. At least try to shoot for nine—the sweet spot of sleep. Getting less than six hours of sleep has been linked to weight gain.

2. The best answer is A. Annual checkups, plus regular dental care, are a must. An annual physical can detect any problems when they're still treatable. Regular dental care and teeth cleaning prevent gum disease, which is nasty. Bad bacteria can head to the heart and cause major problems. So floss daily and get twice-yearly teeth cleanings (or at least yearly).

3. The best answer is C. If you eat balanced fruits and vegetables daily, the stronger your resistance to disease, the more efficient your digestion, and the more control you have over your weight. Always pair servings of fruit or vegetables with a protein and a fat. This combo keeps blood sugar steady, hunger at bay, and your fat-burning mechanisms activated.

4. The best answer is A. Most scientific evidence still backs the recommendation of 2 quarts a day. The minimum limit increases when you engage in strenuous exercise or physical exertion. Also, tea, alcohol, juices, and other flavored beverages don't count—water is what you need. A quick tip is to divide your body weight in half. The number equates to the minimum ounces of water you should drink daily. For example, if you weigh 140, you need 70 ounces of water a day, or roughly nine 8-ounce glasses. The science on hydration is pretty clear: The more water you drink, the greater your weight loss. I carry a favorite water bottle with me at all times, which helps me drink more water through the day. I have a goal of refilling it five times a day so I know I have had enough water.

5. The best answer is A. I can't say enough good stuff about exercise. It's a miracle worker for a great body, lasting weight control, energy, sexual vitality, great health, and longevity. Don't think you need hours and hours of exercise, either. You need quality over quantity. An eight-minute workout that's focused and intense is more effective than an hour workout done too lightly or haphazardly. Diversify your workouts, too, with different programs; boot camp, running, yoga, and so forth. Whatever you do, have fun. The more fun you're having, the better it is for you!

6. The best answer is B. Most people don't eat enough protein. Protein helps build muscles and burn fat. It tames your hunger and keeps you feeling full, especially when you eat it in combination with carbohydrates and fat.

7. The best answer is A. You've probably heard that drinking some wine a few times a week is good for your heart and circulation. True, but it's also associated with a higher risk of breast cancer. Too much alcohol through the week will also make it hard for you to lose body fat, especially that stubborn cellulite. You have to weigh the pros and cons.

8. The best answer is A. Great health is less about what you weigh; it's more about your body composition. Having under 20 percent body fat means you're in great shape. Be careful about going lower than 15 percent, however. That's too low for women, and can be dangerous. It may interfere with your menstrual cycle and cause other health concerns.

9. The best answer is C. Stress levels vary from person to person, and stress will always be present in our lives. It's how you handle and manage it that counts. What's superstressful for me might be only mildly upsetting for you. Stress forces the body to churn out a hormone called cortisol. When chronically elevated, cortisol can cause an accumulation of fat inside your belly. This leads to obesity, health problems, and diabetes. The Badass plan, with its workouts and protein-carb-fat nutrition, is a great stress reducer.

10. The best answer is A. Sugar is really worse than too much dietary fat, because it creates all sorts of metabolic havoc in your body, from blood sugar disturbances to obesity. Give it up!

11. The best answer is B. Smoking will kill you! As I mentioned, I used to be a heavy smoker and I know how hard it is to quit. Honestly, though, nothing is more important to long-lasting health than quitting smoking. 'Nuff said.

12. The best answer is A. Sex is great, but in this day and age, it can kill you if you're not practicing it safely—and with a monogamous partner.

13. The best answer is A. Illicit or "recreational" drugs such as marijuana, cocaine, heroin, and meth will ruin your life and health. So will the abuse of prescription drugs such as painkillers. Get off 'em.

14. The best answer is B. People who are happy, optimistic, and satisfied with their lives live longer and healthier. Tons of research studies bear this out.

15. The best answer is C. To paraphrase an old rhyme: All work and no play make Jill a dull girl. Make time for fun in your life. It harmonizes your body, mind, and soul. Get out and play, and you'll do your health and happiness a world of good.

HOW DID YOU DO?

□ **MORE THAN TEN "BEST" ANSWERS**

Good for you! You are a true Badass health inspiration. Keep making all those smart choices every day. Change in areas where you fall short, and work on improvement.

□ **SEVEN TO NINE "BEST" ANSWERS**

You're on your way to being Badass, but you need to push a little harder. Depending on your answers, you might need to exercise more or harder, cut back on health-damaging behaviors like smoking or drinking, or tweak your nutrition to include more veggies.

□ **LESS THAN SIX "BEST" ANSWERS**

Whoops, you're falling short of the Badass lifestyle. Take charge of your health behaviors now to avert the consequences later. But, beginner Badass, I believe in you: The fact that you were brave enough to take this quiz means you're ready to commit to keeping your body strong and healthy.

EVALUATE YOUR BODY COMPOSITION

Weight scales can't differentiate between muscle and fat pounds. So it might be difficult for some women to know if they're truly overweight. Example: Two women of the same height can each weigh 150 pounds, and one can carry 30 percent body fat and look obese, while the other can have 20 percent body fat and look fit and toned. At 150 pounds, she's firm, lean, strong, and healthy. What she weighs on the scale doesn't really matter. What matters is her *body composition*.

Body composition refers to your percentage of body fat in relation to your percentage of muscle. It's a great overall sign of how healthy you are, as well as indicator of the nutrition and exercise choices you make.

Many techniques are available to analyze your body composition, some fairly simple and others quite complex. For example:

• The **skinfold technique** measures fat just under your skin. As many as ten sites may be measured, although the combined measurement of the abdomen, triceps, chest, and thigh skinfolds is usually enough for an accurate reading. Skinfolds are measured by a set of calipers, a device that pinches up folds of fat away from the underlying muscle tissue. The measurements are plugged into a formula that calculates body fat and lean mass percentages.

The accuracy of the skinfold technique depends on the skill of the person performing the measurements and the number of sites measured. For best results, it's advisable to have your skinfolds measured by a skilled technician, perhaps someone at a local gym or a nurse at your doctor's office. Use the same person each time too. And note that the skinfold technique does not work well with very obese people. Most calipers are usually not large enough to measure their skinfold thicknesses.

• A **bioelectrical impedance scale**, which resembles a bathroom scale, is an easy way to test yourself at home. These scales are inexpensive too—under $50—and you can purchase them at stores such as Target or Walmart.

You simply step on the pad, and the device measures your body composition instantly. It then displays your weight, body fat, total body water, and muscle. These devices are based on the principal of bioelectric impedance, in which an undetectable electric impulse sent through the body is measured as it goes through fat, muscle, and water. A faster signal means you've got a nice amount of muscle on your body. That's because water conducts electricity, and muscle just happens to be approximately 70 percent water. Fat, on the other hand, doesn't contain much water, so it "impedes," or resists, the conduction.

These devices, however, are typically less accurate for people who are obese or very lean.

• Considered the most accurate form of body fat testing, **underwater weighing** positions you in a chair suspended from a scale. After exhaling, you're dunked in a tank of water and required to hold your breath for about ten seconds while your weight under water is measured. The entire procedure is repeated several times. The three heaviest readings are averaged and put into a set of equations to figure out your percentage of body fat. Besides being a hassle, this method is less accurate for women, due to our wide variations in the amount of fat-free mass (bones, muscle, and other nonfat tissue). If you're interested in having this done, check with the sports or health department at a local university. Your doctor may have some sources too.

- There are a few **"low-tech"** tests you can do that I like. One of the simplest methods is take your waist circumference using a nonelastic tape measure. Wrap the tape around the top of your hipbones but without sucking in your tummy. There shouldn't be any slack in the tape either. If your waist measures greater than 35 inches, this suggests that you've got too much body fat, and you may be at a higher risk for heart disease.

You can also assess your body fat distribution by the waist-to-hip ratio (WHR). Using a tape measure, measure your waist at the smallest point—at or near your navel. Then measure your hips at their widest point. Divide your waist circumference by your hip circumference. Let's say you have a 30-inch waist and 40-inch hips. Your waist/hip ratio is 0.75. Under 0.8 is ideal; 0.8 to 0.85 is borderline; and above 0.85 is a risk factor for heart disease and diabetes.

- Or just use the **Jeans-o-Meter!** Slip on your favorite pair of skinny jeans—the ones that got too tight a while back—to see how they're fitting. Having trouble squeezing in? Odds are, you need to start incinerating body fat and developing superfit muscle.

Experts say that for great health and low risk for disease, try to maintain a healthy body fat percentage. The chart below gives you a range to shoot for, based on your activity level. You'll look and feel better if you stay at the lower end of that range.

Here's my final word on this: I know there are a lot of you who like numbers and value accuracy. If you're part of that crowd, by all means use some of the high-tech or low-tech methods to get your body measured, and compare it to the chart. I'm not a doctor or an exercise physiologist. I don't even play them on TV. But I know when someone's too fat. If you want me to tell you whether you have a high body fat percentage, just strip down to your bra and underpants. I'll take a look, and I'll be honest. Only kidding—you can do this yourself.

Body Fat Percentages for Women

Physical Condition	Range
Essential fat (minimal amount of body fat required for health)	10 to 13%
Athletic women	14 to 20%
Fit women (women who work out regularly and are fit)	21 to 24%
Average or lightly active (deemed acceptable for women)	25 to 32%
Obese (increased risk for weight-related illness such as high blood pressure, heart disease, diabetes, gallstones, osteoarthritis, and some cancers)	32% and higher

Source: American Council on Exercise (ACE)

POLICE YOUR PORTIONS

The final *P* in PREP isn't so much about your body or weight; it's about getting into a habit that helps your shape: policing your portions. On the Badass plan, weighing and measuring food really important. It helps you calculate just the right amount of protein, carbs, and fat you need for fat burning and muscle building. Yes, I know. It sounds like a pain to have to do this, and I offer one plan in which you do not have to weigh and measure. But I can assure you, if you want a sexy body and you want it fast, you've got to do some extra work, at least initially, to get it.

You'll need the following tools:

• Measuring cups (1 cup, 1/2 cup, 1/3 cup, and 1/4 cup sizes)
• Measuring spoons (1 tablespoon, 1 teaspoon, 1/2 teaspoon, 1/4 teaspoon)
• A food scale to help you weigh items that can't be measured in cups, such as meat, poultry, and fish.

After measuring and weighing all your foods initially, you'll be able to eyeball your portions (such as when dining out) without having to slap everything on the food scale.

ONE MORE THING: TAKE MY PLEDGE

Right now, I want you to make a . . .

COMMITMENT TO YOURSELF

Look over this pledge and place a star next to each statement. At the bottom, sign your name and date it. Post your pledge where you can see it every day—on your fridge or bathroom mirror or in your car.

———— I am 100% committed to following the Badass plan.

———— I will "show up" for myself for 21 days of this program and do exactly what the plan recommends.

———— I will get rid of tempting foods in my house, and I will replace them with nutritious ones.

———— I will prioritize my health and fitness from this day forward.

———— I will make body-honoring choices, day by day.

———— I agree that the plan is a lifestyle that I'm developing, not something I pick up and put down when I need it.

———— I understand that to take care of my body is to nurture the most valuable physical resource I have.

Signature: _____ Date: _____

Make this 21-day promise to yourself, and make it non-negotiable—no matter what happens in your life. Just 21 days. I know you can do it.

Of course, when I say 21 days, I don't want you to stop there. I want you to follow this way of living on a daily basis, well into the future.

But if you at least make the 21-day pledge to yourself, you'll love the results—in how you feel, mentally and physically, and in how you look. Congratulations on taking the first step!

As you and I go through this program together, I want you to periodically check your progress against your benchmarks. Have you dropped pounds? Have you shaved off body fat percentages? Do you look leaner in the mirror? Have you noticed that you've developed some attractive muscle? Are you controlling your portions and feeling nice and full? Are you feeling more confident and empowered?

Answering yes to any of those questions is powerful motivation for sticking to the plan and changing your lifestyle. If your resolve ever starts to slip, look at how far you've come from those benchmarks, and there's no way you'll turn back.

CHAPTER 4

Booty Foods

WE WOMEN DO A lot to look good on the outside. We pluck our eyebrows, color our hair, get our bikini lines in order, and slather on skin creams and makeup. But when it comes to the inside, many of us let ourselves go. We put crap in our bodies and let them deteriorate through lack of use.

I'll use the analogy of a car engine to explain what I'm talking about. Put sugar in the gas tank and you'll crack the engine. By contrast, put high-octane gas in the tank and your car will run better and longer the car. The human body is the same: the higher the quality of fuel you ingest, the longer you'll be able to run without costly maintenance and the longer it'll be before you break down for good. On the highway of life, you want to zip along like a well-tuned Ferrari, running on quality fuel.

You get that fuel from the right kind of nutrition.

MEET THE MACROS

If you haven't met, let me introduce you to the *macronutrients,* or "macros," for short: protein, carbohydrates, and fat. Everything you eat, from cereal in the morning to a steak for dinner, is made up of macros. This "trifecta of success" provides energy, measured as calories, to maintain life. There are also *micronutrients* in food: vitamins, minerals, and phytochemicals. They don't give you energy, but they help your body metabolize and use the macros. Without macronutrients, we'd starve to death, and without micronutrients, we'd suffer deficiency diseases and poor health and eventually die from malnutrition.

At every meal and snack on the Badass plan, you're going to eat a precise balance of the three macros, which in result will give you a good balance of your micros. Let me give you an overview.

PROTEIN

Of all the macros your body needs to develop firm muscle, protein is king. Why? Because it's an absolute must for building and maintaining all your body's structures. I'm not just talking about muscles, either. I'm talking about tendons and ligaments, blood vessels, brain, organs, skin, your immune system—just about everything. As old cells naturally die off, protein is constantly needed to renew and repair them. If brand-new protein from your diet isn't coming in on a regular schedule, body structures can start to break down.

Protein is a supreme fat burner. Some quick background: proteins, carbohydrates, and fats are measured in terms of their "thermic effect," which refers to how many calories it takes to burn them off. Sugary carbs and fats have around a 3 percent rate; this means it takes 3 calories to burn off 100 calories of these foods. Natural carbs like fruits and veggies have a 20 percent rate (it takes 20 calories to burn off 100 calories of these foods.) Proteins, at 30 percent, have the highest thermic effect of food (TEF), which is why protein is a fat-burning food.

Most of the protein on the Badass plan is animal protein. It's my position that animal protein is an important part of the human diet when balanced correctly, and is definitely a key to getting a firm body.

I know what you're thinking: What about plant-based proteins such as beans, legumes, soy foods, and so forth? These proteins are acceptable, but some of them are high in carbs, while others (such as soy foods and alternative meats like veggie burgers) are often processed, which leads to limited muscle development, and they may do nothing to help eliminate booty fat and cellulite.

A confession: I was a vegetarian for eight years, but at age 20 I started eating meat again, and I haven't looked back. It's one of the reason I was able to put lean muscle on my body. So don't mess with my animal protein. If you try to take steak away from me, you might as well lock me up.

CARBOHYDRATES

Carbohydrates are simply the sugars and starches in our food. The body burns carbs as fuel. The brain also runs off carbs. Have you ever felt draggy and moody? I know I have. This is because your body might be running low on carbohydrates. Carbs include grains, cereals, breads, fruits, and vegetables. They contain essential vitamins and minerals plus fiber and plant nutrients that are vital for health and disease prevention.

Carbs come in two forms: simple and complex. Simple carbohydrates are found naturally in fruits, dairy products, and processed foods such as breads and many packaged foods. They're also found in refined sugars, such as table sugar, that are used in sweet foods. Complex carbohydrates, on the other hand, are found in grains, potatoes, beans, and vegetables.

Carbs can be troublemakers. If you eat too many, you'll get fat. When we eat carbs, the body secretes the hormone insulin in response. Insulin activates enzymes in fat tissue; those enzymes stimulate the body to hold on to fat and pack it away. When insulin levels decline, fat is released and burned. So the worst possible diet is one that's high in carbohydrate, because the body makes fat from carbohydrates and lots of it. That's why you can't eat a lot of carbs and expect to lose weight and get a nice, sexy ass.

I've carefully calibrated the Badass plan to make sure you eat enough carbs for energy, but at levels that keep your body in a fat-burning mode. And I balance carbs with protein and fat for the very best results.

FAT

I love peanut butter, especially on top of my scrambled eggs (no, it's not yucky; the taste is amazing, really!). I love bacon, too, sizzling right next to those eggs. And I eat nicely marbled red meat at times. Yes, some experts still feel that low-fat eating is supposedly important for health, the responsible thing to do, but this view is changing.

I firmly believe that we all need to shift back to eating more fat, including the much-demonized saturated fat. I'm not talking about fatty junk foods or man-made fats like trans fats, but fresh meats and fats such as nut and seed butters, butters, and some cream. These foods are nutritional gold mines.

Surprised? Take a look at all the good things about fat:

1. Fat helps control your hunger. The first purpose of fat is to slow down the rate at which food goes into your bloodstream. The net effect is that you feel satisfied, and any urges to eat more are delayed. If you eat your meals and snacks with fat, you'll need less food than you think. Fat is a natural appetite suppressor!

2. Fat is a carrier for certain vitamins. Several essential vitamins are transported through the body by fat molecules—namely, vitamins A, D, E, and K, also known as the fat-soluble vitamins.

3. Fat makes food taste good. For example, butter is yummy on vegetables (and on popcorn, of course). Greens and salad veggies come to life in oil-based salad dressings, and fresh berries in rich cream is one of life's most scrumptious treats.

The thinking is that fat makes you fat is wrong. There's little evidence that eating fat makes you put on weight. Fat is not fattening. So, fat? Fear not.

I'M A BADASS!

After having her first baby, Amanda, 35, put her body and health on hold and focused on raising her little daughter. Between being a mom, preparing meals, and caring for the house, she didn't feel she had time to watch her weight, and her days felt crammed. She had never really worked out or dieted, so of course the pounds were creeping on, especially around her tummy and thighs. She was starting to feel uncomfortable in her body and disguised herself in her husband's oversize sweats and T-shirts.

When her daughter turned two, Amanda realized she could no longer use "I just had a baby" as an excuse, and she didn't want to be a mom who couldn't keep up with her kids.

I suggested that she follow one of my plans that would ease into better nutrition, with fresh veggies, fruit, and protein, and she could still learn how to balance all the macros for great results.

Talk about results. Here's the big reveal: Amanda lost 15 pounds in the first 21 days. How cool is that?

One of the best things she learned was the importance of making time for herself to eat right and exercise. When she did that, she was much happier and so was her family—which is the most important thing, after all.

PRIMO, ACCEPTABLE, REALLY TERRIBLE MACROS

Macros rule, for sure. But some are better than others, and some are downright bad. I further classify the macros like this:

PRIMO FOODS

These are "whole" foods found in their natural state—no processed crap. They don't have labels or multiple ingredients, either. Examples are:

Proteins. These include meats (beef, pork, lamb, veal, and so forth), poultry; fish, shellfish, eggs, and egg whites.

Non-starchy Vegetables. This category includes broccoli, cauliflower, peppers of all kinds, asparagus, lettuce and other greens, green beans, yellow beans, cabbage, summer squash, cucumbers, tomatoes, radishes, onions, zucchini, and many more. These foods are low in calories, high in fiber, and loaded with nutrition.

Fruits. Fruits are full of nutrients and fiber, plus they provide energy in the form of carbohydrates to power daily activities, including exercising. All types of fruits in whole form are allowed on my plan.

Fats. You get to eat a wide variety of fats on my plan. They give you energy, help your body burn fat, and lubricate your joints. Fats make you happy, too—they're a terrific mood lifter. They also tell your body when you're full and prevent you from overeating. The Badass Fats Choices list on page 72 gives you many options; primo fats such as nuts and seeds are excellent choices because they contain natural fats, fiber, and excellent nutrition.

For your first 21 days, I want you to choose "primo" foods only.

ACCEPTABLE MACROS

There are foods you can pick that are healthy in moderation and with deliberate purpose, but your progress might slow down if you eat too many of them. Examples are dairy products such as milk and cheese and starchy foods like sweet potatoes and natural grains. There are limited benefits in adding dairy foods to your diet; they can be a good combo item but contribute to extra fat gain if not careful. Plus, a lot of people can't stomach the lactose in dairy foods and suffer digestive problems. Most of the nutrients you get from dairy you can get easily from other sources, including canned salmon, broccoli, and green leafy veggies. As for starches, choices like legumes and grains are healthy, but they're carbs. Carbs kick up insulin. You don't want that happening, since insulin interferes with the breakdown of fat and drives fat right into storage. When you eat a balance of carbs, insulin stays in line.

REALLY TERRIBLE MACROS

No matter how good we try to be, there are times when we women turn a little naughty, calling back the guy we know is wrong for us, just because he's good in the sack. Well, "really terrible macros" are like that: tempting but bad for us. I'm talking about junk food here: anything that comes in a box, foods with long lists of ingredients on the label, fast foods, lunch meats, soy products (soy tends to increase estrogen, a fattening hormone), sodas, alcohol, and anything with sugar dumped into it, natural or imitation.

"Really terrible macros" are also known as processed foods. They are loaded with additives, preservatives, flavorings, dyes, processed fats, refined sugar, artificial sweeteners, sodium, and all kinds of gunk and junk. Your body is just not designed to handle these foods, and they will make you fat and unhealthy. Your muscles crave high-quality, primo foods and will respond best when fed the best possible food choices. Put the best fuel into that beautiful body of yours, and it will take you to the highest level of fitness and performance.

That said, I'm a realist, and I know there are times when you want some of these foods. It's okay. I for one like to treat myself to a cupcake every once in a while. Later on, I'll show you how to do some controlled cheating that won't throw your eating plan out of whack. But for best results, you want to avoid the really terrible macros.

PRIMO

Animal meats

Veggies

Fruits

Nuts and seeds

ACCEPTABLE

Dairy

Natural grains and starches

REALLY TERRIBLE

Commercial brand-label foods with long lists of ingredients, additives, and chemicals including breads and pastas.

Alternative meats/proteins such as soy burgers, vegetable burgers, and textured meat protein

Sweets (sugar-containing foods that can be used later on cheat days)

Alcohol (can be used later on cheat days)

FOOD COMBINING, THE BADASS WAY

The "ideal" meal or snack on the Badass plan combines the ideal nutrients—protein, carbohydrate, and fat—in the ideal proportions. So every time you plan a meal or have a snack, make sure it features all three: protein for muscle development and repair, carbs for energy, and fat for appetite control.

My mixed meals approach tips the scales toward a beautifully defined, well-sculpted body and booty. Combining the macros helps keep your blood sugar levels stable. If your blood sugar is in check, you energy levels are high throughout the day, and your ability to burn fat for fuel is much greater. And as I mentioned, fat also plays roles in both fat burning and muscle building, along with general health and emotional well-being.

NOW ABOUT THOSE BOOTY FOODS...

I just went over some general nutrition info on protein, fat, and carbs. Now let's dig into protein, carbohydrates, and fat from the booty-fat-burning side of the equation.

The specific macros you eat throughout the day play a part in how well you shape up your butt. During this program, you're going to learn to pick macros—I call them booty foods—that will burn this stubborn fat right off your booty, thighs, tummy, arms, and elsewhere. You'll get to eat a variety of healthy, satisfying foods, but booty foods play front and center on the Badass plan.

BOOTY PROTEINS

Your derriere is just like any other muscle group in that it needs protein to firm up. To support this process, you're allowed measured amounts of protein at meals. Here are your best choices:

FISH

For my clients I usually recommend fish first and poultry second. Most of my meals go between these two meats because they help me stay leaner. Fish slow-releases protein into your muscles after you eat it. Your body therefore stays in a muscle-building mode around the clock. The omega-3 fats in fish such as tuna and salmon are fat-burning fats, too. Fish also raises levels of a hormone called leptin. Produced by fat cells, leptin governs fat storage by switching your body into fat-burning mode.

CHICKEN AND TURKEY

Poultry is a fantastic source of protein that supports the development of body-firming muscle. Turkey, in particular, contains tryptophan, a substance used by your body to make serotonin—a mood-enhancing, muscle-relaxing, antistress substance. Enjoy turkey, and you're less likely to indulge in sugary excesses and stress eating.

PORK

Drumroll, please: You can eat pork on this plan. Pork is a fat burner! A 2012 study in the journal *Nutrients* reported that people who followed a diet on which pork was the chief protein source were able to change their body composition to more body-firming muscle and less ugly fat. In other words, their shape changed for the better: skinnier waistlines, thinner lower bodies, and less body fat all over. Yay, *nutrients!*

BEEF

Attention, beefophiles: You don't need to give up your beloved red meat. You aren't going to die with a T-bone in your mouth. I know that meat has a bad reputation for being a fatty food, and many people are cutting it out of their diets. And yes, it's high in saturated fat. Don't worry, you need some saturated fat in your diet to boost a little of that fat-burning testosterone.

Beef is loaded with iron, which carries oxygen in your blood and transports it to your muscles and other organs. You need adequate blood flow to support fat burning.

Beef is also packed with several other nutrients that support your quest for a badass body, including the B vitamins. These nutrients are involved in muscle repair after exercise, production of red blood cells, and protein synthesis, all of which help build muscle tissue. We know from studies that people who eat beef lose more weight than those who don't eat beef.

Another plus: beef protects muscle tissue. The more muscle you've got, the higher your metabolism. The net effect: more fat burning, better weight control. More to come on this issue!

That said, if your doctor has told you to cut back on saturated fat, be picky when it comes to the beef you plop on your grill or skillet. My favorites are the eye of round, sirloin tip, bottom round, top sirloin, and 95 percent lean ground beef. These cuts tend to be lower in saturated fat.

EGGS

I can't start my day without eggs. I eat them every morning, with the yolks, because they're loaded with protein that is well absorbed by the body. And they taste great when you prepare them properly.

About the yolk. Far too many cholesterol-challenged folks toss the yolk aside like yesterday's news. A study at the University of Connecticut tested the cholesterol reaction of 25 men and 27 women to an egg diet (640 milligrams a day of additional cholesterol) or a non-egg diet (0 milligrams daily of cholesterol). The cholesterol in yolks didn't raise the nasty LDL cholesterol particles that influence heart disease. Bottom line, you can welcome eggs back into your diet.

Eggs burn belly fat, along with fat all over the body. A 2009 study published in the *Journal of Nutrition, Health & Aging* reported that people who weight-trained and increased their intake of eggs had some pretty impressive changes in their physiques: more muscular legs and abs and less fat in those places. I live for this kind of study. Eggs rule!

WHEY PROTEIN AND RECOVERY SHAKES

On certain of my plans, you're going to be drinking my Recovery Shakes, one or two times a day. These shakes are made with a near-magical protein called whey.

A natural, complete protein derived from cow's milk, whey is a superior protein source. I love it because it helps supply the building blocks of muscles—amino acids—for muscle repair and growth. Whey is also loaded with leucine, a fantastic amino acid that helps burn body fat.

The best time to drink a Recovery Shake is within 10 minutes of exercising, immediately after your workout is complete. Don't wait! There's a lot of research to show that taking whey protein plus some carbs after workouts increases muscle growth. The combo of whey and carbs enhances the body's ability to absorb amino acids, getting them into the muscles, where they impact growth.

If you have a dairy intolerance, it's okay to substitute an alternative protein powder, such as hemp or pea protein.

Hip Advice: Enemies of a Badass

Just as eating the right foods can cause your body to burn fat, eating the wrong foods can bring the fat-burning process to a screeching halt. Those foods include sugar, excessive sodium (salt), processed foods (those with commercial brand labels), and alcohol. Here's a close look:

Sugar. Get off sugar! Remember, it's a "really terrible macro." When you eat sugar and sugar-containing junk, your body uses it as energy, rather than tapping into its fat stores for fuel. You're sabotaging your own fat-burning efforts. It doesn't take a lot of sugar to do this. Even a small piece of chocolate will upset the fat-burning process and be turned right into body fat. I'm talking about all kinds of sugar, not just the white stuff. Avoid the following for now: table sugar, syrups, honey, molasses, brown sugar, jams, jellies, candy, desserts, ice cream, and baked goods—anything you'd classify as a "sweet" is on the blacklist. Be honest with yourself.

Sodium. A little salt is fine, but too much causes a couple of problems related to weight gain. First of all, salt can cause your body to retain water. This skews your true weight loss results on the scale, and it causes cellulite. Second, high consumption of salt causes digestive problems. When your digestive system isn't working up to par, expect to experience constipation and faulty absorption of food and nutrients. As a result, your metabolism slows down and fat is not burned as quickly. This will make you put on weight.

The best way to manage salt in your diet is to avoid processed and packaged foods and get into the habit of eating eat fresh, whole foods that you cook yourself. Do not add table salt to your meals. Instead, get creative with herbs and spices. Sauté meats and veggies in fat-free, no-salt-added chicken broth or wine, or use your barbecue grill.

Dairy. A lot of us can't handle dairy because it can cause bloating, cramps, or embarrassing gas "leaks." It also causes chronic inflammation in the body. Know your body here, and cut out dairy if you can't tolerate this "acceptable" macro. Almond milk is a great substitute.

Alcohol. Ease back on this "really terrible macro" . . . it's full of sugar. It also elevates estrogen abnormally, a situation that creates and worsens cellulite. If you want to include alcohol, use it as a carb, make it sparse, and understand that it will limit your progress more than anything else.

BOOTY FATS

My program emphasizes two types of fat: saturated fat and monounsaturated fats (MUFAs; I call them moo-fas). Because you'll be eating muscle-building protein from mostly animal sources, you'll be taking in some saturated fat. Don't go bonkers on me; hear me out. Saturated fat is important for maintaining testosterone levels. Testosterone is a male hormone, but we women have a little of it, and that's good. In our bodies, it helps burn fat and keeps us a little hornier than usual—two great reasons to befriend this hormone. So basically, we want to supply our bodies with the raw material to build a little testosterone, and that raw material is saturated fat.

As for moo-fas, they can actually reduce belly fat, including the so-called visceral fat packed around your vital organs, which has been linked to a variety of diseases, including diabetes, breast cancer, heart disease, and dementia.

Recent studies indicate that moo-fas are more readily burned for muscle fuel than other types of fat. Plus, moo-fas are great for exercisers. They spare the use of muscle glycogen for energy—a benefit that means you can work out longer and burn more fat in the process. You'll get your moo-fas from almond butter, avocados, and nuts. Don't forget, too, that fats fill you up and keep you satisfied between meals.

You don't get to load up on fats on the plan, but you'll eat just enough to keep you full and happy. Here are your choices:

BACON

With a straight face, I'm going to declare bacon a diet food. I eat it and cook with it almost every day. Bacon is such a great background for so many foods. A little goes a long way. I love that smoky, sweet flavor. As a fat, it keeps you full and satisfied. It's a great source of saturated fat in order to fortify testosterone levels in your system. This works, believe me. Now you have an excuse to eat bacon. But there's a caution: eat it responsibly, and not to the exclusion of plant-based fats such as avocados and nuts. Bacon is great but not the ideal fat for feeling full and satisfied with your meal.

NUTS

Nuts are concentrated packages of protein, vitamins, and moo-fas. Talk about a near-perfect food. Eaten with a protein and a carb, nuts make a great snack. All types of nuts are included on my program. There's some saturated fat in nuts, so you've got some butt-burning power packed in every crunchy bite.

ALMOND BUTTER

Here's my favorite moo-fa: almond butter. Anything almond is fabulous in my book. Almond butter is a super source of minerals, including potassium, which is lost in sweat and needed to prevent muscle cramps. I love blending almond butter into my Basic Booty Recovery Shake. Consider almond butter one of the top fat choices for your meals and snacks.

If you don't care for almond butter (are you nuts?), it's okay to substitute peanut butter—my other top favorite—and other nut butters such as cashew or walnut.

AVOCADOS

I don't think I could live without avocados, a huge source of moo-fas. Avocados are also high in fiber, a nutrient in food that has been shown to help zap thigh and butt fat. At 3 grams of dietary fiber per serving, the avocado has the highest fiber content of any fruit, ounce for ounce.

In addition, the avocado contains other essential nutrients, such as potassium for electrolyte balance, vitamin C for immune function and tissue repair, vitamin E for antioxidant protection and blood cells, vitamin B6 for brain function and red-blood cell formation, and magnesium for muscle contraction.

The mighty avocado is also a belly fat burner—a fact that has been substantiated by research. You can't find a better all-around body-shaping food than the avocado, and it's so versatile—it can be eaten plain or used in a ton of different recipes.

BOOTY CARBS

You know it, I know it: low-carbing ain't easy—at first. On the Badass plan, you'll detox from carbs, and then you won't crave them as much. Your body will start using its fat for energy. Of course, you do get to eat certain carbs, such as fruit carbs, which are normally not allowed on low-carb diets. You also can enjoy veggies and certain starchy carbs like sweet potatoes. I've programmed enough fruits and veggies into this plan that you won't be victimized by relentless cravings for all things sweet and starchy.

Hip Advice: No Artificial Sweeteners Either!

Artificial sweeteners really irk me. They can make you fat—even the occasional diet soda. Fake sweeteners cause many of the same reactions that regular sugar does, because the receptors on your tongue and in your stomach can't discern between real sugar and fake sugar. So artificial sweeteners only trick the brain into craving more sweets and more sugar and throw your blood sugar levels out of balance. Also, our bodies weren't designed to process chemicals and other artificial ingredients. When you ingest one, the body doesn't know exactly what to do with it. So what it does is surround that mystery chemical with fat and tuck it away someplace you'd probably rather not have it.

One of the worst artificial sweeteners is aspartame. When aspartame breaks down in the gut, methanol is formed. You'll find methanol in antifreeze and rocket fuel, among many other applications. The body deals with it by dismantling it into waste products that include formaldehyde, a carcinogen that morticians use to embalm dead bodies. *Really?*

FRUIT CARBS

Eat fruit. I've seen so much evidence that adding fruit to the diet helps you lose weight and stay full and satisfied. Fruit is nature's candy and really the best food you can eat to placate our natural desire for sweets. It's a terrific source of fiber and provides the right balance of carbs in my meal plans.

One of my favorite fruits is apples. I eat apples almost every day with my breakfast because they're slow-burning fruits, meaning that the energy they yield stays with you a long time. This is because they contain pectin, a type of fiber that digests slowly and promotes weight loss. Pectin stops glucose from being absorbed quickly by the body, so we avoid fat storage and sugar cravings.

Oranges get burned up faster but pack higher levels of nutrients, including a whopping dose of vitamin C, which helps your body use hormones for fat burning. In addition, vitamin C creates skin-firming collagen and strengthens the soft-tissue matrix under that skin to make your lower body resistant to cellulite. Oranges also have diuretic properties. They help you shed retained water, which exaggerates the dimpling effect of cellulite.

Berries are superlow in carbs and high in fat-burning fiber. They also have been shown in studies to help your body use insulin more effectively. Insulin tends to be a fat-storing hormone, so you don't want it lazily hanging around in your blood without doing its job (shuttling glucose into cells for energy). Your body may be less sensitive to insulin, which helps you convert sugar into energy.

The nutrients in these berries trigger leptin formation and release from fat cells. The berries also contain carnitine, which assists muscle metabolism—required for burning fat. There are many varieties of berries from which to choose—all fun and delicious—from raspberries to strawberries to blackberries.

Let's move on to grapes. These natural sweet treats get slammed a lot. Critics say grapes are too high in natural sugars to be of any use in a weight loss program. I disagree; research shows that grapes are rich in a certain class of antioxidants called phenolics, which increase thermogenesis in the body; this refers to the generation of heat after you eat a meal. The heat increases your calorie and fat burn. The way I see it, grapes are fat burners. So what if they're a little higher in sugar than a lot of fruits? Combining a dream diet with reality surely must allow for grapes!

While I'm on the subject of fruit carbs, let me add that fruit juices are not allowed. Fruit juices zip through your digestive system; the sugar and carbs in them are likely to be deposited as fat. By contrast, eating fruit in its whole, natural form helps slow down the release of natural sugars in the bloodstream. Those sugars are less likely to be stored away as fat, especially when you eat fruit with protein and fat.

Hip Advice: No Beans About It

You might wonder why my diet doesn't allow beans and most legumes (at least not for the first 21 days). While very healthy, these vegetables contain lectins, which are highly suspect plant substances. Lectins can mimic the effect of hormones—a side effect that can lead to weight gain. They also contain enzyme blockers that screw with the body's ability to digest protein. That's something we don't want, since protein is such a fabulous fat burner.

VEGGIE CARBS

You can eat certain vegetables to your heart's content: mainly green leafy vegetables like spinach, broccoli, lettuce, and any low-calorie veggie. There's evidence that vegetables keep fat-forming estrogen in line, so that you also prevent your butt from spreading any more than it has. Protective chemicals in these foods are responsible. These foods are great sources of vitamin A, which boosts immunity, helps lower cholesterol, controls diabetes, speeds weight loss, and fights digestive problems.

Leafy green vegetables are high in calcium, a mineral that helps keep you slender. Calcium boosts weight loss by inhibiting the production of calcitriol, a hormone that tells cells to generate more fat. Eat salad as much as you want. Mix it up with kale, baby bok choy, and other leafy greens. You don't have to bore yourself to death with iceberg lettuce (which is low in nutrients) all the time in your salads!

Researchers suspect that the antioxidants contained in fruits and vegetables play an important role in warding off abdominal fat. Examples of such antioxidants include beta-carotene, found in carrots and squash, and vitamin C, found in oranges and strawberries.

Hip Advice: Fiber, Estrogen, and Your Butt

If your butt is larger than you want, that means you may have plentiful supplies of the female hormone estrogen in your body. Estrogen promotes the deposit of fat cells in your butt and thighs—and is one of the worst triggers of cellulite.

A high-fiber diet helps decrease estrogen levels by whisking this fat hormone out of your body through the digestive system. Technically, high fiber means about 26 grams of fiber a day—an amount that in research has been showed to burn lower body fat. You can get ample fiber by eating lots of fruits and vegetables. Both food groups are included on this diet.

There are foods that will promote estrogen in your body—and make your butt bigger. They include soybeans and soy products, tofu (bean curd) and tempeh, all of which are high in estrogens. Alcohol has the same effect. Don't eat or drink this stuff if you want a badass body.

EXTRAS

I mix coconut water with a good whey protein power for my Recovery Shakes. I drink them after my most intense workouts—usually three to four times a week—to instigate fat burning and muscle toning.

Also, don't be concerned about your meals being bland. On this diet you can add unlimited amounts of herbs and spices as long as they have minimal salt and don't contain added sugar. Stay away from most sauces, but dry rubs and spices are always welcome.

You can also include dates to get your sweet fix. Dates are as sweet as candy, and one of the healthiest foods you can pop in your mouth. They're packed with more than 60 percent natural sugar in addition to protein, fibers, starch, and fat. Vitamins A, B, and C are also present in dates. The minerals in dates include iron, sodium, calcium, sulfur, and phosphorus. Dates act as diuretics too, countering ugly bloat. Just limit them: one or two a day are enough to curb your sweet tooth and can count as carbs in your overall macronutrient balance.

Hip Advice: Booty Foods at a Glance

Here's the list of booty foods. Post these in your kitchen where you can see them, and choose them often when you plan meals.

BOOTY PROTEINS
Fish
Chicken
Turkey
Pork
Beef
Eggs
Whey protein powder

BOOTY FATS
Nuts/seeds
Nut butters/seed butters
Avocados

BOOTY CARBS

Green leafy vegetables

Veggies

Apples

Berries

Oranges

Grapes

GO GRAZY

Using a big selection of foods, you get to eat six times a day: three meals and three snacks—in other words, you'll "graze." There's solid proof that grazing, or spreading your calories out throughout the day, can keep you trim and fit by cutting down on the amount of food that's converted into fat. There's a cool little study published in the *Journal of the American College of Sports Medicine,* which found that volunteers who ate multiple meals through the day had less body fat than those who ate most of their calories at dinner. Your body can process only so much food at a time, so if you eat too many calories at once, the excess might get packed away as fat.

Try not to skip any of your six eating times, either. If you go more than five hours without eating, your body might respond as if it's starving, even though you know you'll eat again. But your body "thinks" differently and decelerates your metabolism to save calories. The next time you have a meal or snack, your body might store those calories as fat, since the body is stocking up for going without food again. So feel free to eat between main meals, and take advantage of grazing.

Can't squeeze in six mealtimes a day? It's okay to eat three times a day if you're time-crunched. I'll show you how later. The Badass Plan is flexible.

Booty foods, along with other primo macros, automatically switch on the body's natural fat-burning mechanism and help you lose weight and get a bad, sexy ass. If you're feeling uncertain about how and when to eat them, don't worry. I'll give you the skinny in upcoming chapters.

Hip Advice: Coffee

You can drink coffee, but at certain times. Coffee is an appetite suppressant—and I want you to eat—so drink it after your meals. Have one cup then, and no more until your next meal. Also, don't drink coffee after 4:00 p.m. It can keep you awake. I want you to sleep well, because sleep helps you recover and feel energized for the next day. Plus, sleep-deprived people have trouble losing weight because poor sleep negatively affects hormones that regulate fat burning. Coffee is also a diuretic that can flush your body of important nutrients you need to maintain a Badass body.

If you do drink coffee, have it black, without sugar or cream. Sugar can be addictive, and cream is considered a fat. You're allowed fat on my plan, but cream in your coffee could compromise your total fat intake for the day.

For best results, try to reduce your intake of coffee and any other caffeine-containing beverages.

PART 2

PUT IT BEHIND YOU

CHAPTER 5

Step-by-Step Meal Planning:
Your Nutritional Blueprint

LOSING FAT AND GAINING muscle should be fun! But too often diets are known for their boring predictability and bland choices, rather than for their taste and variety. Not here. You'll get to eat a lot of different delicious foods—and six times a day. If you feed your body well and often, and don't sit on your butt inhaling a box of cookies, it will do wonderful things for you. Let the fun begin.

In Part 1, I showed you the basic concepts of my program—how and why it works, the balance of protein, carbs, and fat, the importance of booty foods, and what you can expect. Now it's time to put all of this into motion by planning your meals, eating the proper foods, and making important day-by-day changes in your lifestyle.

First, I'm going to ask you to stick to the program faithfully for just 21 days if your goal is to lose weight, gain muscle, and get a better body. That's just a mere three weeks out of your life! At the end of 21 days, see how you feel and how you look. Are your clothes fitting better? Have you lost weight? How's your energy level? Do you feel excited about the changes taking place in your body?

After 21 days, you can certainly loosen up a bit on the diet and learn how to introduce some occasional "cheats" in your menus. Or you can repeat those three weeks over and over again until you get right down to the beautiful body and butt you want. I will emphasize: *If you continue on the straight and strict path, you'll get the full benefits of the program—faster.*

I'm going to bet that you repeat the three weeks. Why? Because you're going to feel healthier, more energetic, and more mentally vibrant than you've felt in a long time. And you'll start loving the way you look.

The Badass plan is a way of life, not just a diet. You'll learn in the first three weeks how to balance your foods and what foods are better for you. Afterward, you'll be able to incorporate it into a lifetime change of eating habits. This is designed to set you up for success for life, not just for three weeks out of your life.

How can I be so sure? I have heard many, many stories from people who have done my program who say that after even the first week, the changes they've made just felt so good, and their bodies kept getting leaner and tighter with every passing day, thanks to this very powerful food and exercise plan.

Give yourself every chance to succeed. You deserve no less, and I know you'll love the results so much that you'll want to follow this program permanently.

Let's dig in.

STEP 1: Decide Which Plan to Follow

Everyone comes to my program with different requirements and goals, which is why I personalize the diet for four different types of dieters: the *Minimalist*, the *Modifier*, the *Gainer*, and the *Maintainer*. Each is described below.

THE MINIMALIST

This plan is very basic and is designed to help you get started and maintain simplicity. Unlike the other plans, it does not require to you weigh and measure your foods. Weighing and measuring will give you much better results, but if you're not ready to commit to that, I advise that you start out on the Minimalist plan.

It's designed for flexibility—and for the person wants to dip her toe in the pool of my eating plan and guesstimate food portions. You'll still get to lose body fat, but not as quickly or efficiently as you might on another plan. How much muscle you add depends on your workout habits. The more you exercise, the more muscle development you'll gain. You'll eat primo foods exclusively on this plan.

Select the Minimalist plan if one or more of these criteria apply.

- You are interested mostly in reducing body fat.
- You need a more flexible approach that does not involve weighing or measuring portions.
- You aren't sure whether you're a Modifier, Gainer, or Maintainer. If you don't find yourself a precise match to any particular plan, start with the Minimalist.

THE MODIFIER

The Modifier plan is engineered strictly to help you see and feel change right from the get-go, and it is effective for anyone who wants to shed extra pounds fast. You must weigh and measure your foods if you want the best results. Don't be surprised if you drop 15 pounds or more in 30 days.

The Modifier plan has the lowest amount of fat of the four diets; this means it's also the lowest in calories. That way, your body starts to utilize its own "extra storage" faster than the other plans. This is a great plan if you want to get in bikini shape for the beach and the summer months.

Like the Minimalist, the Modifier plan requires that you eat primo foods—pure and natural food choices. It's also a great plan for athletes in sports for which they need to get lean to make weight.

Select the Modifier plan if one or more of these criteria apply.

- You have 40 percent body fat or higher, or are 30 pounds or more overweight.
- You have a lifestyle that is currently sedentary, with very little activity on the job or with exercise.
- You work out, but usually not intensely and three times a week or less.
- You need to get lean quickly for health and cosmetic reasons, or to make weight for an athletic competition.
- You have goals to rapidly lower your body fat, with a minimal gain in body mass.

THE MAINTAINER

Maybe you're close to your weight loss goal, plus you want to build more body-glorious muscle and finally get a tight booty. If either of these sounds like you, you'll follow the Maintainer plan. It also is designed to keep your body fat at a minimum. You'll eat clean, wholesome foods, with allowances for some extra variety in food choices. You have to weigh and measure your foods.

This plan is also for a woman who wants to put on some curvy, sexy muscles. Basically, this means that while your weight looks good on a scale, it makes for a discouraging picture when you get naked and see you're still as soft as the Pillsbury Doughboy, with hardly a trace of definition. In fact, as a skinny-fat person (that is what I was), you may have more fat cells on your body than a lot of your friends who are overweight.

Select the Maintainer plan if one or more of these criteria apply.

- You have 20 to 30 percent body fat.
- You train three to seven times a week, usually at a higher intensity.
- You would like to decrease your body fat.
- You would like to increase your body mass (muscle) percentage more rapidly than a Modifier.

THE GAINER

This plan is for someone who needs to gain more mass, such as an athlete in a "bulk" cycle or a person who's doing an intense training program already, such as a marathon runner or triathlete.

On the Gainer plan, you get to eat the most food of all four plans. This approach won't make you fat, but will put on lean mass for the look and performance you want. Plus, you get to enjoy a wide variety of foods. Weighing and measuring your foods is key for getting results.

Select the Gainer plan if one or more of these criteria apply.

- You have less than 15 percent body fat.
- You are highly active, with an intense workout schedule.
- You train two hours daily or more (approximately ten hours or more of training a week).
- You are close to your ideal body composition, but you'd like to put on additional lean muscle.
- You would like to increase or maintain your body fat percentage.
- You would like to increase your body mass (muscle) percentage more rapidly than a Modifier or Maintainer.

As you follow the Badass plan, you might go through several or all of these plans, depending on where you are with your goals or how your body has changed. If you start off as a Modifier and get close to where you want to be, you can merge into the Maintainer plan, for example. Or if you're very active and want to build some sexy muscle, you can follow the Gainer plan. That's the beauty of this program: you can individualize it according to your goals and body aesthetics.

Take me, for example. I mostly follow the Maintainer plan now, since I'm within my body composition goal and am very active. When I trained for NASCAR, however, I put myself on the Gainer plan in order to fuel myself properly and put some oomph into my performance. I was doing two pit practice or training sessions a day of two hours each, plus my regular workouts. I needed more food to meet the energy demands of pit crewing. The Gainer plan helped me gain muscle, keep my body fat percentage, and increase my performance. Once I was finished with NASCAR, I went back on the Maintainer diet.

For CrossFit training and competitions, I flow through every one of these plans, as the schedule below shows you.

Then, for a national weightlifting competition, I followed the Modifier plan for two weeks. It allowed me to reduce my overall body weight so that I could compete in a specific weight class. That plan pared off body fat without reducing my lean mass to get me to my optimal performance weight for competition. In August, I follow the Minimalist plan, after being strict for most of the year due to competition and training.

Hip Advice: 12 Months of Christmas

How I Flow Through the Four Plans

In the course of a year, I use each plan. Because I'm an athlete, I base my plan selection on my competition goals for the year. Here's what my year typically looks like.

January: Maintainer. I'm prepping for the CrossFit Open Qualifier but don't want to put on too much mass for the competition so that I can be fast and strong. I do regular exercise classes and additional lifting—plus a little extra for competition preparation.

February: For the CrossFit Open Qualifier competition, I follow either the Maintainer or Gainer, depending on my workouts. I train five or six times a week, plus a little extra for the competition needs.

March: Gainer. My goal is to put on strength and mass. I train five to seven times a week, approximately 10 to 15 hours a week.

April: I may flow from Gainer to Maintainer and some Minimalist when needed.

May: For the CrossFit Regionals competition, I follow the Maintainer plan. It helps me perform fast, but doesn't make me too heavy.

June: Maintainer and Minimalist. I'm training five to seven times a week, approximately 10 to 15 hours a week.

July: To prepare for the CrossFit Games and US Weightlifting Nationals Competition, I follow the Modifier plan for a month. After the competition, I may switch to the Minimalist plan. I relax my training a bit.

August: Minimalist. I kick back to enjoy the rest of my summer and relax on weighing and measuring my food. But I stay true to the system and always balance my meals. I train in a single CrossFit class, boot-camp-type class, running, or yoga. Overall, I work out about four to six times a week. I don't go to extremes; I just try to mix things up and have fun with my workouts.

September: Maintainer. I'm back in the saddle and eating for strength. My training schedule is still four to six times a week, but I'm pushing my effort higher.

October: Gainer. I've worked off any extra pounds I might have gained since August. My goal now is to build muscle. I increase my training to five times a week, devoting an hour and a half to each workout session. I'm lifting heavy weights, training for endurance, and doing hot yoga.

November: I switch to the Modifier plan for three weeks to cut weight and make my weight class, but without losing strength. My training tapers off about two weeks out from my competition. The week of my competition, I follow the Maintainer plan to keep up power and strength.

December: Maintainer. Here I'm gearing up for the American Weightlifting Open competition. After the competition, I follow the Minimalist plan until January.

So you see, the Badass plan is flexible and designed to work with your body and your goals throughout an entire year and a lifetime. It doesn't always have to be dialed in, but going strict with a plan occasionally helps keep measurements in perspective while being a Minimalist.

PERSONALIZE THE PROGRAM

The plan I will initially follow is: _____

STEP 2: Figure Out How Much Food You Should Eat

Getting the body you want is like building a house. You need a strong foundation and sturdy walls; all the marble countertops and sparkly finishes don't matter one iota if the house is about to collapse.

The foundation of my diet is primo foods with a little bit of acceptable foods, along with properly prepared, nutritionally dense booty foods. Once you build your foundation with these foods, you can start building your walls—something you'll do with nutrient combinations I call bricks.

A brick is comprised of a specific quantity of protein, carbohydrate, and fat, and is used to put together your meals. You'll eat a certain number of bricks at each of your meals and snacks. The number is based on two factors: 1) the diet you're on—Minimalist, Modifier, Maintainer, or Gainer; and 2) your frame size, determined by your height. Think about it: A woman who is five feet ten inches is definitely going to require more food than someone who is five feet two. You'll learn how to tailor the plan to your individual height profile.

Here's how to determine your height profile:

Frame 1 (Mighty): 4′10″ to 5′2″
Frame 2: (Force) 5′3″ to 5′6″
Frame 3: (Power) 5′7″ to 5′10″
Frame 4: (Bold) 5′11″ to 6′
Frame 5: (Confident) Over 6′

The number of bricks you eat each day looks like this:

Frame	Minimalist	Modifier	Maintainer	Gainer
Frame 1 **Mighty**	See the guidelines on page 80.	8–12 bricks	9–13 bricks	11–14 bricks
Frame 2 **Force**	See the guidelines on page 80.	11–13 bricks	11–15 bricks	14–17 bricks
Frame 3 **Power**	See the guidelines on page 80.	12–14 bricks	13–17 bricks	14–18 bricks
Frame 4 **Bold**	See the guidelines on page 80.	13–16 bricks	14–18 bricks	15–19 bricks
Frame 5 **Confident**	See the guidelines on page 80.	15–20 bricks	16–20 bricks	16–22 bricks

The meal plans are built according to this blueprint. This system will take a little getting used to, but before long, it will become second nature—and the key to making long-term changes in your diet and nutrition.

Nothing worthwhile is without effort. The majority of the "work" with this program is on the front end. Once you're a few days into it, the Badass plan becomes exceptionally easier to comprehend and apply.

PERSONALIZE THE PROGRAM

My frame is _____.

Each day, I'll eat a total of _____ bricks.

> ### I'M A BADASS
>
> Allison, age 26, was always a "big-boned" girl and accepted it early on. She had gone on many diets and tried different styles of eating. Some worked, but she always fell off the wagon eventually because of restrictions or complications. Allison decided to attend one of my seminars because she knew that my plans are individualized for different-size frames.
>
> Allison shared the following with me: "The seminar was great! I felt like I finally had the tools that made sense to help me take control of my body. After only a week, I felt so much better! I had more energy and more mental clarity at work. Over the first several weeks, I lost 23 pounds."
>
> Ultimately, Allison was able to maintain a weight and body composition that made her feel confident and sexy and healthy for her frame.
>
> She added, "Your program really helped me discover my body I knew I had—and I was never hungry!"

STEP 3: Know How Many Bricks You'll Eat for Each Meal and Snack

Meals and snacks are made up of multiple bricks, which often give you a range. Usually, you'll plan your meals at the lower end of the range. But if you feel hungry, you can adjust your bricks to include the number at the higher end of the range. Refer to the following chart to figure out how many bricks you'll eat for breakfast, lunch, dinner, and snacks.

MODIFIER

Meal	Frame 1 MIGHTY	Frame 2 FORCE	Frame 3 POWER	Frame 4 BOLD	Frame 5 CONFIDENT
Number of Bricks					
Breakfast	1–3	2–3	2–3	2–3	3–4
Snack	1	1–2	1–2	1–2	2–3
Lunch	2–3	2–4	2–3	3–4	3–4
Snack	1	2	2	2	2–3
Dinner	3	3	3–4	4	4–5
Snack	0–1	1	1	1	1
Total	8–12	11–13	12–14	13–16	15–20

MAINTAINER

Meal	Frame 1 MIGHTY	Frame 2 FORCE	Frame 3 POWER	Frame 4 BOLD	Frame 5 CONFIDENT
Number of Bricks					
Breakfast	2	2–3	2–3	2–4	3–4
Snack	1	1–2	2–3	2	2–3
Lunch	2–4	3–4	3–4	4–5	4–5
Snack	1–2	2	2	2	2
Dinner	2–3	2–3	3–4	3–4	4–5
Snack	1	1	1	1–2	1
Total	9–13	11–15	13–17	14–18	16–20

GAINER

Meal	Frame 1 MIGHTY	Frame 2 FORCE	Frame 3 POWER	Frame 4 BOLD	Frame 5 CONFIDENT
Number of Bricks					
Breakfast	2–3	3–4	3–4	3–4	3–5
Snack	1	1	2	2	3
Lunch	2–3	3–4	4–5	4–5	3–5
Snack	2	2	2	2	2
Dinner	3–4	4–5	3–4	3–4	4–5
Snack	1	1	1	2	2
Total	11–14	14–17	14–18	15–19	16–22

MINIMALIST

On the Minimalist plan, meals and snacks are put together by combining a primo protein, a primo carbohydrate, and a fat to make a breakfast, lunch, dinner, or snack. There are no bricks involved, only the combination of the three macros. Minimalist meal plans begin on page 80, where you'll learn how to put it together.

STEP 4: Understand the Macronutrient Composition of a Brick

Depending on whether you're a Modifier, Gainer, Maintainer, or Minimalist, the macronutrient composition of your bricks will differ slightly. For example:

The macronutrient assignment per brick for **Modifiers** is as follows:

1 brick =

7 grams of protein

5 grams of carbohydrate

1.5 grams of fat

In food terms, that brick looks like:
- 1 large hard-boiled egg (7 grams of protein)
- 10 medium strawberries (5 grams of carbohydrate)
- 3 raw almonds (1.5 grams of fat)

The macronutrient assignment per brick for **Gainers** and **Maintainers** is as follows:

1 brick =

7 grams of protein

5 grams of carbohydrate

4.5 grams of fat (MAXIMUM, meaning eat enough fat to make you happy and full but this measurement is your max. Don't eat more than this, but you can eat less if necessary.)

In food terms, that brick looks like:
- 1 large hard-boiled egg (7 grams of protein)
- 5 medium strawberries (5 grams of carbohydrate)
- 9 raw almonds (4.5 grams of fat)

PERSONALIZE THE PROGRAM

On my program, one brick is _____ grams of protein; _____ grams of carbohydrate; and _____ grams of fat.

STEP 5: Include Recovery Shakes and Meal Replacements

As part of my program, you can enjoy Recovery (where noted) and Meal Replacement Shakes. Each has a different purpose, but both will help you achieve your goals.

Recovery Shakes are meant to be taken immediately after your workout. Your body works hard during exercise. Muscle tissue is broken down. Nutrients are lost. Muscle fuel is expended. Muscle hormones are compromised. All of these need to be replenished and fortified fairly quickly after a workout.

The Recovery Shake to the rescue: Have this shake immediately after your workout. It will replenish your body with everything that was used up. Science shows that having a recovery beverage—one that combines protein and carbohydrates—after exercise creates a hormonal environment conducive to muscular development and fat burning. Specifically, hormones such as growth hormone, testosterone, and thyroid hormones are all bolstered when you supercharge your worked-out body with these key nutrients. Timing is everything.

Recovery Shakes do not contain any fat, however. Fat slows down the absorption of protein and carbs. Because you want those two macros to get to your muscles as fast as possible, my Recovery Shakes are fat-free. See the delicious recipes for you beginning on page 223.

The Meal Replacement Shake is a filling concoction of protein, carbohydrate, and fat. It is designed to substitute for any breakfast, lunch, dinner, or snack. What I love about this option is that it's perfect for anyone with a busy schedule—a student with no time to cook, a mom who's having a tough time making three full meals a day, or a career women who barely has time for lunch. You just put a few key ingredients in a blender, and in seconds you're sipping on a delicious meal. (My delicious recipes start on page 227.)

Meal replacements can help you on your journey to a knockout body. In a recent study, it was found that one of the most important predictors of successful weight loss is the use of meal replacements, plus weekly exercise activity. If you've never used meal replacements, I encourage you to start because they help you control your brick portions and help you lose body fat.

Hip Advice: Are You a Three-Meals-a-Day Person?

I'm often asked if you have to eat six times a day. No, not really. If you prefer to eat three meals a day—breakfast, lunch, and dinner—you can certainly do that. This means that you'll take your snack bricks and fold them into those three meals. The key is really to eat your allotted number of bricks for the day. You can distribute them among three meals and three snacks a day, or just have three meals. These plans are extremely flexible and designed to work with your schedule and desires.

THE BRICKS LIST

You don't have to count grams of protein, carbs, or fats. You don't even have to count calories. All you have to do is count bricks, and that's easy.

The following list of foods is organized into proteins, carbohydrates, and fats. Within each group, you can see what constitutes one brick, and you can use these lists to build your meals.

The foods I've listed here give you with a variety of choices to help you plan your meals. You just need to keep track of how many bricks you have at each meal or snack—and ensure that you have a balance of protein, carbohydrate, and fat each time. At first, trying to absorb all of this information can be difficult, but trust me, in a week or two, you'll have it mastered, and you'll know instinctively how much food makes up a brick.

BADASS PROTEIN CHOICES

The Primo and Acceptable Protein Measurements for Minimalists, Modifiers, Maintainers, and Gainers

Foods from this group are divided into three categories: eggs and protein powder; land proteins (animal proteins); and sea proteins (seafood).

Food	1 Brick Measurement
Eggs and Protein Powder	
Egg, whole	1 large
Egg whites	2 large
Egg substitute	¼ cup
Land	
Beef	1 ounce
Beef, ground	1 ounce
Chicken breast	1.5 ounces
Chicken, ground	1.5 ounces
Deli meat	1½ slices
Duck	1.5 ounces
Ham	1 ounce
Lamb	1 ounce

Pork	1 ounce
Pork, ground	1.5 ounces
Turkey breast	1.5 ounces
Turkey, ground	1 ounce
Veal	1 ounce

Sea

Catfish	1.5 ounces
Crabmeat	1.5 ounces
Flounder/sole	1.5 ounces
Lobster	1.5 ounces
Mahimahi	1.5 ounces
Salmon	1.5 ounces
Sardines	1.5 ounces
Scallops	1.5 ounces
Swordfish	1.5 ounces
Shrimp	1.5 ounces
Tuna steak	1.5 ounces
Tuna—canned in water	1.5 ounces

THE REALLY TERRIBLE PROTEINS FOR MINIMALISTS, MODIFIERS, MAINTAINERS, AND GAINERS

Avoid: Any alternative protein, such as tofu, soy burgers, soy sausages, and textured vegetable protein; fatty processed meats such as bologna or salami. (Deli meats are fine.)

BADASS CARBOHYDRATE CHOICES

The Primo Carbohydrate Measurements for Minimalists, Modifiers, Maintainers, and Gainers

Non-starchy vegetables and fruits are all classified as primo carbohydrates. You'll want to obtain most of your primo carbs from the non-starchy vegetables list first, with the fruit list second.

Food	1 Brick Measurement
Non-Starchy Vegetables	
Artichoke, cooked	¼ cup
Asparagus, cooked	9 spears
Bean sprouts, raw	1 cup
Beet greens, cooked	1 cup
Bok choy, cooked	2 cups
Broccoli, cooked	¾ cup
Broccoli, raw	1¼ cups
Brussels sprouts	½ cup
Cabbage, cooked	1 cup
Cabbage, raw	1¾ cups
Cauliflower, cooked	1 cup
Cauliflower, raw	1½ cups
Celery, raw	1¾ cups
Collard greens, cooked	½ cup
Cucumber, raw	half
Dill pickle	1 large (5 inches)
Eggplant, cooked	¾ cup
Green beans, cooked	½ cup
Kale, cooked	¾ cup
Kale, raw	3¼ cups
Leeks, cooked	¾ cup
Mushrooms, raw	2 cups
Mushrooms, cooked	¾ cup
Okra, cooked	½ cup
Onion, raw	⅓ cup
Onion, cooked	¼ cup
Peppers, raw	½ cup
Peppers, cooked	½ cup
Radishes, raw	1¼ cups
Salsa	¼ cup
Sauerkraut	1 cup
Spaghetti squash, cooked	½ cup

Spinach, cooked	1⅓ cups
Spinach, raw	4 cups
Swiss chard, cooked	¾ cup
Tomato, raw	1 cup
Tomato sauce	½ cup
Tomatoes, stewed or cooked	⅓ cup
Yellow squash, cooked	1 cup
Zucchini, cooked	1 cup

Fruits

Apple	quarter
Apricot	2 small
Banana	quarter
Blackberries	⅓ cup
Blueberries	¼ cup
Cantaloupe	⅓ cup
Cherries	5
Cranberries, sweet dried	2½ teaspoons
Dates, deglet	1
Figs	2
Grapefruit	⅓ cup
Grapes	¼ cup
Guava	⅓ cup
Honeydew	⅓ cup
Kiwi	half
Kumquat	2
Lemon	half
Lime	half
Mango	¼ cup
Nectarine	half
Orange	quarter
Papaya	¼ cup
Peach	quarter
Pear	quarter
Pineapple	¼ cup

Plum	1
Prunes	2
Raisins	1 tablespoon, or 15 raisins
Raspberries	⅓ cup
Strawberries	½ cup
Tangerine	half
Watermelon	⅓ cup

The Primo and Acceptable Carbohydrate Measurements for Maintainers and Gainers

Food	1 Brick Measurement
Grains	
Barley, cooked	⅛ cup
Buckwheat, cooked	⅛ cup
Bulgur wheat, cooked	3 tablespoons
Grits, cooked	⅛ cup
Quinoa, cooked	⅛ cup
Rolled oats, cooked	¼ cup
Rice, brown, cooked	⅛ cup
Starchy Vegetables	
Beets	¼ cup
Butternut squash	¼ cup
Carrots	⅓ cup
Corn, sweet	⅛ cup
Hubbard squash	¼ cup
Parsnips	¼ cup
Peas, green	¼ cup
Potato, baked	⅓ cup
Potato, boiled	⅓ cup
Potato, mashed	⅕ cup
Sweet potato, baked	⅛ cup
Sweet potato, mashed	⅛ cup
Turnip	½ cup

Beans and Lentils

Black beans, cooked	⅕ cup
Black-eyed peas, cooked	⅕ cup
Chickpeas, cooked	⅛ cup
Kidney beans, cooked	⅛ cup
Lentils, cooked	⅛ cup
Lima beans, cooked	⅛ cup
Pinto beans, cooked	⅛ cup

The Really Terrible Carbohydrates for Minimalists, Modifiers, Maintainers, and Gainers

Avoid these—unless you're having an occasional cheat meal.

Carbohydrates	1 Brick Measurement
Breads and Cereals	
Bagel	quarter
Biscuit	quarter
Bread	¼ slice
Breadstick	half
Cereal, ready-to-eat	⅓ ounce
Corn bread	quarter
Croissant	quarter
Doughnut	quarter
English muffin	quarter
Graham cracker	1
Granola	¼ cup
Muffin	quarter
Pancake	quarter
Pita bread	quarter
Roll, dinner	quarter
Roll, hamburger, hot dog	quarter
Saltine crackers	4
Taco shell	half

Tortilla, flour	third
Waffle	third
White pasta	¼ cup
Whole-grain pasta	¼ cup

Snack Foods

Corn chips	⅓ ounce
French fries	3
Popcorn	2 cups
Pretzels	½ ounce
Tortilla chips	⅓ ounce

Alcohol and Sweets

Beer	4 ounces
Liquor	½ ounce
Wine	2 ounces
Chocolate bar	¼ ounce
Ice cream	⅛ cup

BADASS FATS CHOICES

I separate primo fats into two categories: primo fats for Minimalists and Modifiers and primo fats for Maintainers and Gainers. The difference has to do with the amount of fat: on the Maintainer and Gainer plans, you eat a little more fat than you do on the other plans. Try to choose fats that will satisfy you and that make you feel happy after eating them.

The Primo Fat Measurements for Minimalists and Modifiers

Fats	1 Brick Measurement
Almonds	3
Avocado	1 tablespoon
Cashews	3
Macadamia nuts	1
Peanuts	6
Peanut butter	½ teaspoon
Sunflower seeds	¼ teaspoon

The Primo Fat Measurements for Maintainers and Gainers

Fats	1 Brick Measurement
Almonds	9
Avocado	3 tablespoons
Cashews	9
Guacamole	1½ tablespoons
Macadamia nuts	2
Peanuts	18
Peanut butter	1½ teaspoons
Sunflower seeds	¾ teaspoons

Acceptable Fat Measurements for Maintainers and Gainers

These foods can be used sparingly when you plan your meals, but not on the Minimalist or Modifier plans.

Dairy	1 Brick Measurement
Cottage cheese	¼ cup
Butter	1 teaspoon
Cream cheese	1 tablespoon
Half-and-half	3 tablespoons
Sour cream	2 tablespoons

READING LABELS TO DETERMINE BRICKS

The Really Terrible Macros are generally foods with commercial labels listing a lot of ingredients and additives. If you decide to cheat with one of these foods, it's important to understand how much of that processed food equals one brick. Here's a sample label for a bag of high-protein chips:

Nutrition Facts

Serving Size 1 Bag (32g)
Servings Per Container 8

Amount Per Serving

Calories 120   Calories from Fat 20

% Daily Value*

Total Fat 2g	3%
Saturated Fat 0g	0%
Trans Fat 0g	
Cholesterol 10mg	3%
Sodium 150mg	6%
Potassium 65mg	2%
Total Carbohydrate 5g	2%
Dietary Fiber 0g	0%
Sugars 0g	
Protein 21g	42%

First, read through the label, and look for these major items:

Serving Size: 1 bag
Servings Per Container: 8

Second, check the macronutrient content and do the math:

Protein: 21 grams (Divide this by 7 and you get 3 bricks.)
Fat: 2 grams (Divide this by 4½ and you get approximately ½ brick.)
Carbohydrate: 5 grams (Divide this by 5 and you get 1 brick.)

Be aware of what you're putting into your body, especially when it comes in a box or bag with a commercial label. Brand-label food is in the Really Terrible category for a reason: it's far from the best nutrition you can give your body.

The Condiments List for Minimalists, Modifiers, Maintainers, and Gainers

These are permissible, but please use them sparingly. They pack a lot of empty calories in a little bit.

Carbohydrate Condiments	1 Brick Measurement
Barbecue sauce	1 tablespoon
Cocktail sauce	1 tablespoon
Ketchup	1 tablespoon
Pickle, sweet, such as bread-and-butter	3 slices
Relish, sweet	2 teaspoons
Steak sauce	1 tablespoon
Teriyaki sauce	¾ tablespoon

THE LISTS IN ACTION

Let me give you an example of how to use the lists. Let's say you're on the Modifier plan, and you're a frame 3 (Power). You know you get 2 bricks at breakfast, 2–3 bricks at lunch, 3 bricks at dinner, and 1–2 bricks for each of your three daily snacks.

By consulting the list of foods, you might create a daily menu that looks like this:

Breakfast—2 bricks
2 eggs (14 grams of protein)
½ medium apple (10.5 grams of carbohydrate)
1 teaspoon peanut butter (3 grams of fat)

Lunch—3 bricks
Small baked chicken breast—4.5 ounces (21 grams of protein)
2 cups cooked broccoli/carrot medley (15 grams of carbohydrate)
⅛ avocado (4.5 grams of fat)

Dinner—3 bricks

Small serving of roasted turkey breast—4.5 ounces (21 grams of protein)

2 cups cooked green bean/yellow bean medley (15 grams of carbohydrate)

3 macadamia nuts (4.5 grams of fat)

Snack 1—1 brick

1½ slices deli turkey (7 grams of protein)

⅓ cup grapes (5 grams of carbohydrate)

3 raw almonds (1.5 grams of fat)

Snack 2—1 brick

1½ slices deli turkey (7 grams of protein)

¼ small orange (5 grams of carbohydrate)

3 raw almonds (1.5 grams of fat)

Snack 3—1 brick

Hard-boiled egg (7 grams of protein)

5 medium strawberries (5 grams of carbohydrate)

3 raw almonds (1.5 grams of fat)

Okay, I know you're wondering if you can put together your own plan. Yes, you can! All you really require is determination, and a willingness to alter your eating habits. You're now in control of when and what you eat.

Just as you make a household budget, you have to make an eating plan. Put together your meals for the week, including snacks, and stick to it. Making the proper food choices today, and then a little bit tomorrow, will build a regular routine—one in which you'll start dropping weight, putting on curvy muscles, and of course, getting healthier.

BADASS MEAL-PLANNING TEMPLATE

Here's a great tool I developed to help you with this whole meal-planning thing. Simply fill in how many bricks you'll eat at meals, then write in the protein, carbs, and fats you have. Voilà—you've got your meal plan for the week. I've got you starting on Monday, that lucky diet-starting day, but you can begin on any day you want.

Print this template and save it each week you do a meal plan. Keep it simple and build a new food item each week. Save it as Week 1, Week 2, Week 3, and so on. Once you have a few weeks of meal plans saved, you can rotate them, and your meal plan work is already done for you. You can also rotate a new week for each week of the month, then start over in the beginning of the month. Swap days or weeks with a friend to add a little variety.

DAILY BRICK BREAKDOWN FOR MEAL PLANNING

Week: _____

MONDAY

Meal	Bricks	Proteins	Carbohydrates	Fats
Breakfast				
Snack				
Lunch				
Snack				
Dinner				
Snack				

TUESDAY

Meal	Bricks	Proteins	Carbohydrates	Fats
Breakfast				
Snack				
Lunch				
Snack				
Dinner				
Snack				

WEDNESDAY

Meal	Bricks	Proteins	Carbohydrates	Fats
Breakfast				
Snack				
Lunch				
Snack				
Dinner				
Snack				

THURSDAY

Meal	Bricks	Proteins	Carbohydrates	Fats
Breakfast				
Snack				
Lunch				
Snack				
Dinner				
Snack				

FRIDAY

Meal	Bricks	Proteins	Carbohydrates	Fats
Breakfast				
Snack				
Lunch				
Snack				
Dinner				
Snack				

SATURDAY

Meal	Bricks	Proteins	Carbohydrates	Fats
Breakfast				
Snack				
Lunch				
Snack				
Dinner				
Snack				

SUNDAY

Meal	Bricks	Proteins	Carbohydrates	Fats
Breakfast				
Snack				
Lunch				
Snack				
Dinner				
Snack				

Remember, the Badass plans are designed to teach you a balanced way of eating with an emphasis on food quality in terms of protein, carbohydrates, and fats. *If you feel overwhelmed, take a step back and see the bigger picture.* Your life won't derail if one meal is marginally off. But once you learn my system, you can do it with ease and tweak it any way you want, to adjust it to your lifestyle. Keep at it—those benefits are for life!

For more assistance with meal planning, I've put together sample meal plans in the next several chapters that provide delicious combos of foods, along with scrumptious recipes, to help you enjoy what you eat.

CHAPTER 6

The Badass Meal Plans for Minimalists

THE MINIMALIST PLAN IS designed to help you eat primo macros in the proper combinations and proportions. To keep the plan as simple as possible, use what I call the Badass Plate tool: Just visualize a round dinner plate divided into fourths: one-fourth is for your primo protein, one fourth is for your primo fat and the other two-fourths are for your primo vegetables and/or occasionally fruit. I call this the Badass Plate. As an example: grilled salmon + asparagus + mashed cauliflower + avocado.

As for snacks, simply have smaller portions of primo proteins and carbs and fats than you would for your main meals. Also, depending on your frame size (measured by height), you may want to scale down or scale up your portions of food at breakfast, lunch, and dinner.

Don't stuff yourself, though, or pile food mile-high on your plate (that's no fair!). Eat until you're satisfied and then step away from the plate. There's some trial and error involved here, so watch your results and see how effectively you're trimming down.

With balanced macro choices, even though you're not counting bricks, you'll still burn up fat that's already stored on various parts of your body. The rapid results will give you the motivation to continue losing weight all the way down to your goal.

THE 6 PRINCIPLES OF CHRISTMAS FOR MINIMALISTS

I have 6 simple principles to help you get the best results. If you're unsure of anything, refer to these guidelines.

1. Follow the plan strictly for 21 days. If you cheat or deviate, you have to restart.

2. Do not eat any processed foods, sugary foods, or alcohol for the first 21 days. Generally, eat what is assigned. However, you may substitute a similar protein, carbohydrate, or fat for any macronutrient you don't like. For example, if you don't like broccoli, substitute another primo carbohydrate, such as sautéed kale or bok choy. You don't have to clean your plate, but you must eat a balance of the carbohydrates, protein, and fat. You can't eat just the carbohydrates and be done! When you feel full, stop eating.

3. Plan your meals to include a balance of primo proteins, carbohydrates, and fat with emphasis on Booty Foods. Refer to the chart Hip Advice: Booty Foods at a Glance on page 47 for help in selecting these foods. You do not need to weigh and measure your food. You can replace any meal or snack with a Meal Replacement Shake (see page 227). Use the Badass Plate tool to select your proportions.

4. Eat breakfast within 45 minutes after waking up. This is imperative to jump-start your metabolism. Do not go more than five daytime hours without eating.

5. Have one balanced primo meal within one hour of completing your workout.

6. Drink 8 to 10 cups (64 to 80 ounces) of pure water daily, in addition to coffee and green tea if you drink them. Do not drink any sodas or other naturally or artificially sweetened beverages. No diet soda!

The following seven-day meal plan will show you how to plan your Minimalist menus.

Day 1

Breakfast

2 eggs, scrambled or poached, in a teaspoon of oil

Handful of grapes

Water, green tea, or coffee, with no sugar or milk

Snack

Tuna mixed served on several sliced tomatoes

3 almonds

Lunch

Chicken Wraps (page 200)

Water, green tea, or coffee, with no sugar or milk

Snack

Recovery Shake (recipes start on page 223)

Dinner

1 filet mignon grilled or pan-fried

Steamed asparagus

Fresh pineapple chunks

3 almonds

Water (no caffeine after 3:00 p.m.)

Snack

1 slice deli turkey, 2 small apricots, 9 almonds

Day 2

Breakfast

3 eggs scrambled with chopped tomatoes and chopped red bell pepper

Spoonful of peanut butter

1 plum

Water, green tea, or coffee, with no sugar or milk

Snack

1 slice deli turkey, handful of raisins mixed with a handful of almonds

Lunch

Sweet Tuna Salad (page 200)

Water, green tea, or coffee, with no sugar or milk

Snack

Recovery Shake (recipes start on page 223)

Dinner

Pork chop, grilled or pan-fried, drizzled with barbecue sauce

Cooked Brussels sprouts

Cooked yellow squash

2 scoops peanut butter

Water (no caffeine after 3:00 p.m.)

Snack

Heaping spoonful of tuna served on a sliced tomato

3 almonds

Breakfast
2 hard-boiled eggs

Cereal bowl of mixed berries: strawberries, blueberries, and blackberries

Almond butter

Water, green tea, or coffee, with no sugar or milk

Snack
Recovery Shake (recipes start on page 223)

Lunch
Ground beef patty, pan-fried

Stewed tomatoes

3 almonds

Water, green tea, or coffee, with no sugar or milk

Snack
1 slice deli meat (turkey or ham), quarter of an apple with a spoonful of peanut butter

Dinner
Veal chop, covered with tomato sauce

Mixed raw greens, drizzled with balsamic vinegar

2 tablespoons of almond butter

Water (no caffeine after 3:00 p.m.)

Snack
1 hard-boiled egg, quarter of an apple with half a spoonful of peanut butter

Day 4

Breakfast

2 eggs scrambled with 1 slice of ham (chopped)

Grapefruit sections

Handful of mixed nuts

Water, green tea, or coffee, with no sugar or milk

Snack

1 slice deli ham, red bell pepper slices, 5 olives

Lunch

Ground turkey patty, pan-fried

Cooked green beans, sprinkled with crushed almonds

Water, green tea, or coffee, with no sugar or milk

Snack

Recovery Shake (recipes start on page 223)

Dinner

"Spaghetti" and Meatballs (page 209)

Water (no caffeine after 3:00 p.m.)

Snack

1 hard-boiled egg, quarter of an apple with half a spoonful of peanut butter

Day 5

Breakfast

Mexican Omelet (page 194)

Water, green tea, or coffee, with no sugar or milk

Snack

Spoonful of tuna served on sliced tomato

3 almonds

Lunch

Stuffed Tomato with Crab Salad (page 199)

Water, green tea, or coffee, with no sugar or milk

Snack

Recovery Shake (recipes start on page 223)

Dinner

Catfish, baked or grilled, served with a spoonful of cocktail sauce

Creamy Coleslaw (page 216)

Water (no caffeine after 3:00 p.m.)

Snack

Half of a chicken breast, celery sticks spread with a spoonful of peanut butter

Day 6

Breakfast

3 turkey sausage patties

1 nectarine

1 plum

Small handful of almonds

Water, green tea, or coffee, with no sugar or milk

Snack

Recovery Shake (recipes start on page 223)

Lunch

Naked Taco Salad (page 201)

Water, green tea, or coffee, with no sugar or milk

Snack

1 hard-boiled egg, ½ nectarine, 9 almonds

Dinner

Low-Carb Lovers' Pizza (page 212)

18 almonds

Water (no caffeine after 3:00 p.m.)

Snack

1 slice deli ham, red bell pepper sliced, 3 almonds

Day 7

Breakfast

6 egg whites scrambled with cooked mushrooms

Grapefruit sections

Handful of nuts

Water, green tea, or coffee, with no sugar or milk

Snack

Badass Eggs (2 halves) (page 220), raw broccoli

Lunch

Sweet Tuna Salad (page 200)

Water, green tea, or coffee, with no sugar or milk

Snack

Recovery Shake (recipes start on page 223)

Dinner

Grilled salmon with a spoonful of cocktail sauce

Steamed asparagus

18 almonds

Water (no caffeine after 3:00 p.m.)

Snack

1 slice deli turkey, 1 tablespoon raisins, 10 peanuts

I'M A BADASS

Lisa is a stay-at-home mom with two beautiful children. For years, she relied on the "I just had a baby" excuse for being overweight. But the excuse finally got old, and she couldn't rely on it anymore. Lisa was ready to change.

Several of her friends had been on my program—and with great results. Seeing their bodies finally convinced Lisa to get on board.

"The first week was tough," she said. "I had to break some bad eating habits. But I stuck with it, following the Minimalist plan. Before long, I was sleeping better, I had more energy, I was in a better mood around my kids, and my blemished skin improved."

Best of all, after 21 days, Lisa was shopping for new, smaller-sized jeans. She tossed out her old fat pants and put on her new skinny jeans. In fact, Lisa lost four dress sizes in just one month.

"I love the fact that I can fix these meals for my whole family. We're all happier and healthier as a result."

CHAPTER 7

The Badass Meal Plans for Modifiers

I'VE PREPARED THE MODIFIER meal plans to help you design your own daily menus, to show you how to include primo and booty foods in terms of bricks, and to give you lots of variety in food choices. Using these sample meal plans can make everything easier for you, especially as you start out. Later on, you'll be able to plan your own menus in your sleep!

Of course, these plans are only guidelines, so don't let them restrict you. Some people like to eat the same breakfast every day. That's perfectly okay—please do so if you like! If you don't like some of the food choices on the plans, that's okay too. Feel free to substitute the foods you prefer from the lists. And try out my recipes for variety (they're listed in italics in the meal plans). The Badass Recipes start on page 190.

On the Modifier plan, you'll eat primo and booty foods. Your weight loss will be faster, and you'll see your booty get tight and firm faster.

THE 6 PRINCIPLES OF CHRISTMAS FOR MODIFIERS

I have 6 simple principles to help you get the best results. If you're unsure of anything, refer to these guidelines.

1. Follow the plan strictly for 21 days, observing how many bricks you eat daily. If you cheat or otherwise deviate, you must restart the 21 days. You don't have to clean your plate. When you feel full, stop eating, but ensure your macros were balanced for what you ate.

2. Do not eat any processed foods, grains, gluten-containing foods, sugary foods, or alcohol for the first 21 days. This will help your body detox off all that nasty stuff. Choose primo foods and booty foods when planning your meals. Refer to the chart Hip Advice: Booty Foods at a Glance on pages 47–48 for a list of booty foods.

3. Have your breakfast within 45 minutes after waking up. Do not go more than five daytime hours without eating.

4. Have a meal or snack within one hour after your workout, no Recovery Shakes (these are different from Meal Replacement Shakes).

5. Generally, eat what is assigned. However, you may substitute a protein, carbohydrate, or fat for any macronutrient you don't like. For example, if you don't like Brussels sprouts, substitute another non-starchy vegetable carbohydrate. You can also replace any meal with a Meal Replacement Shake (recipes start on page 227).

6. Drink 8 to 10 cups (64 to 80 ounces) of pure water daily, in addition to coffee and green tea. Try to reduce your caffeine intake or cut it out altogether. Do not drink any sodas or other naturally or artificially sweetened beverages. No diet soda! These are considered cheats and are not allowed.

MODIFIER MENUS FOR FRAME 1 (MIGHTY) AND FRAME 2 (FORCE)

The difference between the two frames is that the Force gets to eat 1 extra brick as a snack, and I have noted this in the sample meal plan. Remember too that in each frame, you usually eat a range of bricks. Adjust up and down within that range for your own needs. Feel free to substitute any meal with a Meal Replacement Shake.

Week
1

Day 1

Breakfast—2 bricks

1 egg, scrambled or poached, ½ apple with 1 teaspoon peanut butter

Water, green tea, or coffee, with no sugar or milk

Snack—1 brick

1.5 ounces canned tuna served on ⅓ cup chopped tomato

3 almonds

Lunch—3 bricks

Chicken Vegetable Soup (page 197)

Water, green tea, or coffee, with no sugar or milk

Snack—1 brick for a Mighty

1 hard-boiled egg, ¼ apple with ½ teaspoon peanut butter

Snack—2 bricks for a Force

2 hard-boiled eggs, ½ apple with 1 teaspoon peanut butter

Dinner—3 bricks

4.5 ounces sirloin steak

18 steamed asparagus spears, sprinkled with 3 crushed almonds

1 cup cooked cauliflower

Water (no caffeine after 3:00 p.m.)

Snack—1 brick

1½ slices deli turkey, 2 small apricots, 3 almonds

Day 2

Breakfast—2 bricks
Mexican Omelet (page 194)
Water, green tea, or coffee, with no sugar or milk

Snack—1 brick
1½ slices deli turkey, 1 tablespoon raisins, 3 almonds

Lunch—3 bricks
4.5 ounces canned tuna served over 2 cups mixed greens, ½ cup bean sprouts, and ¼ cup chopped onion,
    and drizzled with 1 tablespoon balsamic vinegar
9 almonds
Water, green tea, or coffee, with no sugar or milk

Snack—1 brick for a Mighty
1 hard-boiled egg, ¼ apple with ½ teaspoon peanut butter

Snack—2 bricks for a Force
2 hard-boiled eggs, ½ apple with 1 teaspoon peanut butter

Dinner—3 bricks
Smothered Pork Chops (page 213)
Water (no caffeine after 3:00 p.m.)

Snack—1 brick
1.5 ounces canned tuna served on ⅓ cup chopped tomato
3 almonds

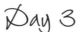
Day 3

Breakfast—2 bricks

2 ounces ham, pan-fried

¼ cup blueberries mixed with ¼ chopped apple

6 almonds

Water, green tea, or coffee, with no sugar or milk

Snack—1 brick

1 hard-boiled egg, ¼ apple with ½ teaspoon peanut butter

Lunch—3 bricks

Texas-Style Chili (page 198)

9 almonds

Water, green tea, or coffee, with no sugar or milk

Snack—1 brick for a Mighty

1½ slices deli turkey, ¼ apple with ½ teaspoon peanut butter

Snack—2 bricks for a Force

3 slices deli meat (turkey or ham), ½ apple with 1 teaspoon peanut butter

Dinner—3 bricks

3 ounces veal chop, pan-fried in 1 teaspoon olive oil, and covered with ¼ cup tomato sauce

2 to 3 cups mixed raw greens, drizzled with 1 tablespoon balsamic vinegar

Water (no caffeine after 3:00 p.m.)

Snack—1 brick

1 hard-boiled egg, ¼ apple with ½ teaspoon peanut butter

Day 4

Breakfast—2 bricks
Mini Quiche (page 195)
Water, green tea, or coffee, with no sugar or milk

Snack—1 brick
1½ slices deli turkey, ½ cup red bell pepper slices, 3 almonds

Lunch—3 bricks
3-ounce ground turkey patty
1½ cups cooked green beans
9 crushed almonds sprinkled on top
Water, green tea, or coffee, with no sugar or milk

Snack—1 brick for a Mighty
Badass Eggs (2 halves) (page 220), 1¼ cups raw broccoli

Snack—2 bricks for a Force
Badass Eggs (4 halves) (page 220), 2½ cups raw broccoli

Dinner—3 bricks
4.5 ounces grilled chicken breast
Zucchini Side Spaghetti (page 218)
Water (no caffeine after 3:00 p.m.)

Snack—1 brick
1 hard-boiled egg, ¼ apple with ½ teaspoon peanut butter

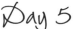

Day 5

Breakfast—2 bricks

4 egg whites, scrambled

2 cups sliced strawberries

12 cashews (doubled since no fat in the eggs)

Water, green tea, or coffee, with no sugar or milk

Snack—1 brick

1.5 ounces canned tuna served on 1 cup chopped tomato

3 almonds

Lunch—3 bricks

Stuffed Tomato with Crab Salad (page 199)

Water, green tea, or coffee, with no sugar or milk

Snack—1 brick for a Mighty

1.5 ounces grilled chicken breast, 8 dill pickle slices, 6 peanuts

Snack—2 bricks for a Force

3 ounces chicken breast, 16 dill pickle slices, 12 peanuts

Dinner—3 bricks

Blackened Whitefish (page 202)

Creamy Coleslaw (page 216)

Water (no caffeine after 3:00 p.m.)

Snack—1 brick

1.5 ounces grilled chicken breast, 2 to 3 celery sticks spread with ½ tablespoon almond butter

Day 6

Breakfast—2 bricks

2 eggs, scrambled

Grain-Free Granola (page 196)

Water, green tea, or coffee, with no sugar or milk

Snack—1 brick

1.5 ounces grilled chicken breast, ½ cup red bell pepper slices, 3 almonds

Lunch—3 bricks

Naked Taco Salad (page 201)

Water, green tea, or coffee, with no sugar or milk

Snack—1 brick for a Mighty

1 hard-boiled egg, ½ nectarine, 3 almonds

Snack—2 bricks for a Force

2 hard-boiled eggs, 1 nectarine, 6 almonds

Dinner—3 bricks

3 ounces ground beef, cooked and mixed with ⅓ cup tomato sauce and ¼ cup cooked onions and
 served over ¾ cup baked eggplant slices

9 almonds

Water (no caffeine after 3:00 p.m.)

Snack—1 brick

1½ slices deli ham, ½ cup red bell pepper slices, 3 almonds

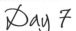

Breakfast—2 bricks

4 egg whites scrambled with ½ cup cooked mushrooms

⅔ cup grapefruit sections

6 cashews

Water, green tea, or coffee, with no sugar or milk

Snack—1 brick

Badass Eggs (2 halves) (page 220), 1¼ cups raw broccoli

Lunch—3 bricks

Sweet Tuna Salad (page 200)

Water, green tea, or coffee, with no sugar or milk

Snack—1 brick for a Mighty

1½ slices deli turkey, 8 dill pickle slices, 6 peanuts

Snack—2 bricks for a Force

3 slices deli ham, 16 dill pickle slices, 12 peanuts

Dinner—3 bricks

"Smoked" Salmon (page 203)

9 steamed asparagus spears

3 almonds

Water (no caffeine after 3:00 p.m.)

Snack—1 brick

1½ slices deli turkey, 1 tablespoon raisins, 6 peanuts

MODIFIER MENUS FOR FRAME 3 (POWER) AND FRAME 4 (BOLD)

The difference between the two frames is that the Bold can eat 2 extra bricks, if desired. Remember, too, that for each frame, you usually eat a range of bricks. Adjust up and down within that range for your own needs. Feel free to substitute any meal with a Meal Replacement Shake (recipes start on page 227).

Week 1

Day 1

Breakfast—2 bricks
2 eggs, scrambled, ⅔ cup grapes, 3 almonds
Water, green tea, or coffee, with no sugar or milk

Snack—1 brick
1.5 ounces canned tuna served on 1 cup chopped tomato, 3 almonds

Lunch—3 bricks
4.5 ounces grilled chicken breast
1½ cups steamed green beans
9 sliced almonds on top
Water, green tea, or coffee, with no sugar or milk

Snack—2 bricks
Egg Muffin Snacks (page 221), ½ apple

Dinner—3 bricks
3 ounces filet mignon
18 steamed asparagus spears
½ cup fresh pineapple chunks
9 almonds
Water (no caffeine after 3:00 p.m.)

Snack—1 brick
1½ slices deli turkey, 2 small apricots, 3 almonds

Day 2

Breakfast—2 bricks

Mexican Omelet (page 194)

Water, green tea, or coffee, with no sugar or milk

Snack—1 brick

1½ slices deli turkey, 1 tablespoon raisins, 3 almonds

Lunch—3 bricks

4.5 ounces canned tuna served over 2 cups mixed greens, 1 cup bean sprouts, and ¼ cup chopped onions
   drizzled with 1 tablespoon balsamic vinegar

18 peanuts chopped over salad

Water, green tea, or coffee, with no sugar or milk

Snack—2 bricks

Egg Muffin Snacks (page 221), ½ apple

Dinner—3 bricks

3 ounces pork chop, grilled or pan-fried, drizzled with 1 tablespoon barbecue sauce

1 cup cooked Brussels sprouts

½ cup cooked yellow squash

1½ teaspoons cashew butter

Water (no caffeine after 3:00 p.m.)

Snack—1 brick

1.5 ounces canned tuna served on 1 cup chopped tomato, 3 almonds

Day 3

Breakfast—2 bricks

2 ounces of ham, pan-fried

Mixed berries: ½ cup strawberries, ¼ cup blueberries

6 crushed cashews topped on fruit

Water, green tea, or coffee, with no sugar or milk

Snack—1 brick

1 hard-boiled egg, ¼ apple with ½ teaspoon peanut butter

Lunch—3 bricks

3-ounce ground beef patty, pan-fried

1 cup canned stewed tomatoes

9 almonds

Water, green tea, or coffee, with no sugar or milk

Snack—2 bricks

3 slices deli meat (turkey or ham), ½ apple with 1 teaspoon peanut butter

Dinner—3 bricks

3 ounces veal chop, covered with ⅓ cup tomato sauce

2 to 3 cups mixed raw greens, drizzled with 1 tablespoon balsamic vinegar

9 almonds

Water (no caffeine after 3:00 p.m.)

Snack—1 brick

1 hard-boiled egg, ¼ apple with ½ teaspoon peanut butter

Day 4

Breakfast—2 bricks

2 eggs, scrambled

⅔ cup grapefruit sections

1 teaspoon peanut butter

Water, green tea, or coffee, with no sugar or milk

Snack—1 brick

1½ slices deli ham, 1 cup red bell pepper slices, 3 almonds

Lunch—3 bricks

4.5-ounce ground turkey patty

1½ cups cooked green beans

9 crushed almonds on top

Water, green tea, or coffee, with no sugar or milk

Snack—2 bricks

Badass Eggs (4 halves) (page 220), 2½ cups raw broccoli

Dinner—3 bricks

Nude Chicken Fajitas (page 207)

Water (no caffeine after 3:00 p.m.)

Snack—1 brick

1 hard-boiled egg, ¼ apple with ½ teaspoon peanut butter

Day 5

Breakfast—2 bricks
Mini Quiche (page 195)
Water, green tea, or coffee, with no sugar or milk

Snack—1 brick
1.5 ounces canned tuna served on 1 cup chopped tomato, 3 almonds

Lunch—3 bricks
Chicken Wraps (page 200)
Water, green tea, or coffee, with no sugar or milk

Snack—2 bricks
3 ounces chicken breast, 8 dill pickle slices, 12 peanuts

Dinner—3 bricks
4.5 ounces catfish, baked or grilled, served with 2 tablespoons cocktail sauce
Creamy Coleslaw (page 216)
Water (no caffeine after 3:00 p.m.)

Snack—1 brick
1.5 ounces chicken breast, 1¼ cups celery sticks spread with ½ teaspoon almond butter

Day 6

Breakfast—2 bricks

3 ounces turkey sausage

1 nectarine

6 almonds

Water, green tea, or coffee, with no sugar or milk

Snack—1 brick

1.5 ounces grilled chicken breast, ½ cup red bell pepper slices, 3 almonds

Lunch—3 bricks

Naked Taco Salad (page 201)

Water, green tea, or coffee, with no sugar or milk

Snack—1 brick

1 hard-boiled egg, ½ plum, 3 almonds

Dinner—3 bricks

Stuffed Peppers (page 210)

Water (no caffeine after 3:00 p.m.)

Snack—1 brick

1½ slices deli ham, ½ cup red bell pepper slices, 3 almonds

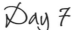

Day 7

Breakfast—2 bricks

4 egg whites scrambled with ¼ cup cooked mushrooms

⅔ cup grapefruit

6 almonds

Water, green tea, or coffee, with no sugar or milk

Snack—1 brick

Badass Eggs (2 halves) (page 220), 1¼ cups raw broccoli

Lunch—3 bricks

Sweet Tuna Salad (page 200)

Water, green tea, or coffee, with no sugar or milk

Snack—2 bricks

3 slices deli turkey, 16 dill pickle slices, 12 peanuts

Dinner—3 bricks

4.5 ounces salmon with 2 tablespoons cocktail sauce

9 steamed asparagus spears

9 almonds

Water (no caffeine after 3:00 p.m.)

Snack—1 brick

1½ slices deli ham, 1 tablespoon raisins, 6 peanuts

MODIFIER MENUS FOR FRAME 5 (CONFIDENT)

Remember that for each frame, you are permitted to eat within a range of bricks (see chart on page 62). Adjust up and down within that range for your own needs. Feel free to substitute any meal with a Meal Replacement Shake.

Week 1

Day 1

Breakfast—2 bricks
Mexican Omelet (page 194)
Water, green tea, or coffee, with no sugar or milk

Snack—2 bricks
3 ounces canned tuna served on 2 cups chopped tomato, 6 almonds

Lunch—2 bricks
Chicken Vegetable Soup (page 197)
Water, green tea, or coffee, with no sugar or milk

Snack—2 bricks
2 hard-boiled eggs, ½ apple with 2 teaspoons peanut butter

Dinner—3 bricks
3 ounces filet mignon
18 steamed asparagus spears
½ cup fresh pineapple chunks
1½ teaspoons peanut butter
Water (no caffeine after 3:00 p.m.)

Snack—1 brick
1½ slices deli turkey, 2 small apricots, 3 almonds

Day 2

Breakfast—2 bricks

Mexican Omelet (page 194)

Water, green tea, or coffee, with no sugar or milk

Snack—2 bricks

3 slices deli turkey, 2 tablespoons raisins, 6 almonds

Lunch—3 bricks

4.5 ounces canned tuna served over 2 cups mixed greens, ½ cup bean sprouts, and ¼ cup chopped onions
  and drizzled with 1 tablespoon balsamic vinegar

9 almonds

Water, green tea, or coffee, with no sugar or milk

Snack—2 bricks

2 hard-boiled eggs, ½ apple with 1 teaspoon peanut butter

Dinner—3 bricks

3 ounces pork chop, grilled or pan-fried, drizzled with 1 tablespoon barbecue sauce

1 cup cooked Brussels sprouts

½ cup cooked yellow squash

9 almonds

Water (no caffeine past 3:00 p.m.)

Snack—1 brick

1.5 ounces canned tuna served on 1 cup chopped tomato, 3 almonds

Day 3

Breakfast—2 bricks

2 ounces ham, pan-fried

Mixed berries: ½ cup strawberries, ¼ cup blackberries

1 teaspoon peanut butter

Water, green tea, or coffee, with no sugar or milk

Snack—2 bricks

2 hard-boiled eggs, ½ apple with 1 teaspoon peanut butter

Lunch—3 bricks

4.5-ounce ground beef patty, pan-fried

1 cup canned stewed tomatoes

9 almonds

Water, green tea, or coffee, with no sugar or milk

Snack—2 bricks

3 slices deli meat (turkey or ham), ½ apple with 1 teaspoon peanut butter

Dinner—3 bricks

Herb-Roasted Lamb (page 214)

2 to 3 cups mixed raw greens with 1 tablespoon balsamic vinegar

Water (no caffeine past 3:00 p.m.)

Snack—1 brick

1 hard-boiled egg, ¼ apple with ½ teaspoon peanut butter

Day 4

Breakfast—2 bricks

2 eggs, scrambled
⅔ cup grapefruit sections
1 teaspoon peanut butter
Water, green tea, or coffee, with no sugar or milk

Snack—2 bricks

3 slices deli ham, 1 cup red bell pepper slices, 6 almonds

Lunch—3 bricks

4.5-ounce ground turkey patty
1½ cups cooked green beans
9 crushed almonds sprinkled on top
Water, green tea, or coffee, with no sugar or milk

Snack—1 brick

Badass Eggs (2 halves) (page 220), 1¼ cups raw broccoli

Dinner—3 bricks

Nude Chicken Fajitas (page 207)
Water (no caffeine past 3:00 p.m.)

Snack—1 brick

1 hard-boiled egg, ¼ apple with ½ teaspoon peanut butter

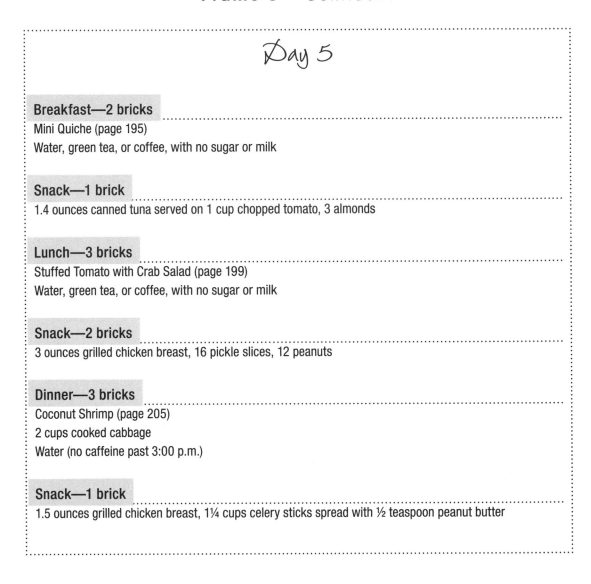

Day 5

Breakfast—2 bricks
Mini Quiche (page 195)
Water, green tea, or coffee, with no sugar or milk

Snack—1 brick
1.4 ounces canned tuna served on 1 cup chopped tomato, 3 almonds

Lunch—3 bricks
Stuffed Tomato with Crab Salad (page 199)
Water, green tea, or coffee, with no sugar or milk

Snack—2 bricks
3 ounces grilled chicken breast, 16 pickle slices, 12 peanuts

Dinner—3 bricks
Coconut Shrimp (page 205)
2 cups cooked cabbage
Water (no caffeine past 3:00 p.m.)

Snack—1 brick
1.5 ounces grilled chicken breast, 1¼ cups celery sticks spread with ½ teaspoon peanut butter

Day 6

Breakfast—2 bricks
2 eggs, scrambled
Grain-Free Granola (page 196)
1 teaspoon peanut butter
Water, green tea, or coffee, with no sugar or milk

Snack—2 bricks
3 ounces grilled chicken breast
1 cup red bell pepper slices
6 almonds

Lunch—3 bricks
Naked Taco Salad (page 201)
Water, green tea, or coffee, with no sugar or milk

Snack—2 bricks
2 hard-boiled eggs, 1 nectarine, 6 almonds

Dinner—3 bricks
4.5 ounces cooked ground beef mixed with ⅓ cup tomato sauce and ¼ cup cooked onions and served over ¾ cup baked eggplant slices
9 almonds
Water (no caffeine past 3:00 p.m.)

Snack—1 brick
1½ slices deli ham, 1 cup red bell pepper slices, 5 olives

Day 7

Breakfast—2 bricks

Mexican Omelet (page 194)

Water, green tea, or coffee, with no sugar or milk

Snack—1 brick

Badass Eggs (2 halves) (page 220), 1¼ cups raw broccoli

Lunch—3 bricks

Texas-Style Chili (page 198)

9 almonds

Water, green tea, or coffee, with no sugar or milk

Snack—2 bricks

3 slices deli turkey, 16 pickle slices, 12 peanuts

Dinner—3 bricks

4.5 ounces salmon with 2 tablespoons cocktail sauce

9 steamed asparagus spears

9 almonds

Water, green tea, or coffee, with no sugar or milk

Snack—1 brick

1½ slices deli turkey, 1 tablespoon raisins, 6 peanuts

I'M A BADASS

Natalie, age 29, took a Boot Camp exercise course from me. Afterward, she decided to get serious about her nutrition, so she went on the Modifier plan.

Her results were certainly ones for the record book.

"In the first month, I lost six pant sizes," she said. "I couldn't believe it. I was happy with how my booty looked, too. I wouldn't say it got smaller, but it sure did get tighter and more lifted."

Natalie has stayed on the plan, moving into different categories depending on her goals at the time.

"I love the program and only eat high-quality balanced macronutrients now. Once you know how simple it is, you can't ignore it."

CHAPTER 8

The Badass Meal Plans for Maintainers

THE MAINTAINER PLAN ALLOWS for a slightly higher amount of fat, and it shows you how to incorporate a few additional food choices into your menus while still taking off pounds.

You have a lot of foods from which to choose, so you're free to create a virtually endless variety of meals. To make it a cinch for you, here are sample meals plans that you can follow exactly or adapt to your own meal-planning preferences.

THE 6 PRINCIPLES OF CHRISTMAS FOR MAINTAINERS

I have 6 simple principles to help you get the best results. If you're unsure of anything, refer to these guidelines.

1. Follow the plan strictly for 21 days, observing how many bricks of each macronutrient you eat at meals.

2. Do not eat any processed foods, sugary foods, gluten, or alcohol for the first 21 days. If you cheat or otherwise deviate, you must restart the 21 days. Choose mostly primo foods and booty foods when planning your meals. Refer to the chart Hip Advice: Booty Foods at a Glance on page 47 for a list of booty foods. Fruit is allowed in its whole. You can replace any meal or snack with a Meal Replacement Shake. You don't have to clean your plate. When you feel full, stop eating.

3. Add in two Acceptable starches (one at breakfast, the other at lunch or dinner), if desired. You can have a little dairy if you want (one dairy a day), but it's optional. A lot

of women can't handle dairy because it causes ugly and uncomfortable bloat. I for one don't do dairy well. Generally, eat what is assigned. However, you may substitute a protein, carbohydrate, or fat for any macronutrient you don't like. For example, if you don't like Brussels sprouts, substitute another non-starchy vegetable carbohydrate.

4. Have your breakfast within 45 minutes of waking up. This is imperative to jump start your metabolism. Do not go more than 5 daytime hours without eating.

5. You can choose to have one Recovery Shake daily on this plan, immediately after completing your workout if it was an intense workout. I've created several shake recipes for you; they begin on page 223. Remember, if you take your Recovery Shake these bricks will count towards your daily brick assignment. Your Recovery Shake must be consumed within 10 minutes of completing your workout, before your cool-down. A Recovery Shake is different from a Meal Replacement Shake.

6. Drink 8 to 10 cups (64 to 80 ounces) of pure water daily, in addition to coffee and green tea. Try to cut back on coffee and caffeine or get off it altogether. Do not drink any sodas or other naturally or artificially sweetened beverages. No diet soda!

THE MAINTAINER MENUS FOR FRAME 1 (MIGHTY)

Remember that for each frame, you are permitted to eat within a range of bricks (see page 62). Adjust up and down within that range for your own needs. Feel free to substitute any meal with a Meal Replacement Shake (recipes start on page 227).

Day 1

Breakfast—2 bricks
Mexican Omelet (page 194)
Water, green tea, or coffee, with no sugar or milk

Snack—1 brick
1.5 ounces canned tuna served on 1 cup chopped tomato, 3 almonds

Lunch—3 bricks
Chicken Wraps (page 200)
Water, green tea, or coffee, with no sugar or milk

Snack—1 brick
Recovery Shake (recipes start on page 223)

Dinner—3 bricks
3 ounces sirloin steak
18 steamed asparagus spears
5 cherries
27 almonds
Water (no caffeine past 3:00 p.m.)

Snack—1 brick
1½ slices deli turkey, 2 small apricots, 3 almonds

Day 2

Breakfast—2 bricks

2 eggs, scrambled

Grain-Free Granola (page 196)

Water, green tea, or coffee, with no sugar or milk

Snack—1 brick

¼ cup cottage cheese, mixed with 1 tablespoon raisins and 9 chopped almonds

Lunch—3 bricks

4.5 ounces canned tuna served over 2 cups mixed greens, 1 cup bean sprouts, and ¼ cup chopped onions and drizzled with 1 tablespoon balsamic vinegar

27 almonds

Water, green tea, or coffee, with no sugar or milk

Snack—1 brick

Recovery Shake (recipes start on page 223)

Dinner—3 bricks

Smothered Pork Chops (page 213)

Water (no caffeine after 3:00 p.m.)

Snack—1 brick

1.5 ounces canned tuna served on 1 cup chopped tomato, 9 almonds

Day 3

Breakfast—2 bricks

2 ounces ham, pan-fried

½ orange

1 tablespoon cashew butter

Water, green tea, or coffee, with no sugar or milk

Snack—1 brick

1 ounce ham, ¼ apple with 1½ teaspoons peanut butter

Lunch—3 bricks

4.5 ounces cooked ground beef mixed with ⅓ cup tomato sauce and ¼ cup cooked onions and served over 1 cup spaghetti squash

27 almonds

Water, green tea, or coffee, with no sugar or milk

Snack—1 brick

Recovery Shake (recipes start on page 223)

Dinner—3 bricks

Nude Chicken Fajitas (page 207)

Water (no caffeine after 3:00 p.m.)

Snack—1 brick

1 hard-boiled egg, ¼ apple with 1½ teaspoons peanut butter

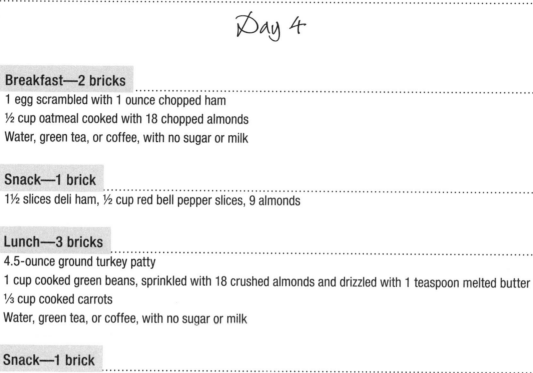

Day 4

Breakfast—2 bricks

1 egg scrambled with 1 ounce chopped ham

½ cup oatmeal cooked with 18 chopped almonds

Water, green tea, or coffee, with no sugar or milk

Snack—1 brick

1½ slices deli ham, ½ cup red bell pepper slices, 9 almonds

Lunch—3 bricks

4.5-ounce ground turkey patty

1 cup cooked green beans, sprinkled with 18 crushed almonds and drizzled with 1 teaspoon melted butter

⅓ cup cooked carrots

Water, green tea, or coffee, with no sugar or milk

Snack—1 brick

Recovery Shake (recipes start on page 223)

Dinner—3 bricks

4.5 ounces grilled chicken breast

1 cup spaghetti squash sauce topped with ⅓ cup tomato sauce mixed with ¼ cup cooked onion

27 almonds

Water (no caffeine after 3:00 p.m.)

Snack—1 brick

1 hard-boiled egg, ¼ apple with 1½ teaspoons peanut butter

Day 5

Breakfast—2 bricks

2 egg whites, scrambled

⅔ cup grapes

6 teaspoons peanut butter (no fat in the eggs so the fat is doubled)

Water, green tea, or coffee, with no sugar or milk

Snack—1 brick

1.5 ounces canned tuna served on ⅓ cup chopped tomato, 6 almonds

Lunch—3 bricks

Spinach Salad (page 201)

Water, green tea, or coffee, with no sugar or milk

Snack—1 brick

Recovery Shake (recipes start on page 223)

Dinner—3 bricks

Turkey Loaf (page 208)

Water (no caffeine after 3:00 p.m.)

Snack—1 brick

1.5 ounces grilled chicken breast, 2 to 3 celery sticks spread with 1½ teaspoons almond butter

Day 6

Breakfast—2 bricks

Mini Quiche (page 195)

Water, green tea, or coffee, with no sugar or milk

Snack—1 brick

1.5 ounces grilled chicken breast, ½ cup red bell pepper slices, 9 almonds

Lunch—3 bricks

Naked Taco Salad (page 201)

Water, green tea, or coffee, with no sugar or milk

Snack—1 brick

Recovery Shake (recipes start on page 223)

Dinner—3 bricks

4.5 ounces cooked ground beef mixed with ⅓ cup tomato sauce sautéed with 1 cup spinach and
   served over 1 cup spaghetti squash

27 almonds

Water (no caffeine after 3:00 p.m.)

Snack—1 brick

1½ slices deli ham, ½ cup red bell pepper slices, 9 almonds

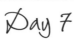
Day 7

Breakfast—2 bricks

2 eggs, scrambled

Grain-Free Granola (page 196)

Water, green tea, or coffee, with no sugar or milk

Snack—1 brick

Badass Eggs (1 half) (page 220)

1¼ cups raw broccoli

Lunch—3 bricks

Sweet Tuna Salad (page 200)

Water, green tea, or coffee, with no sugar or milk

Snack—1 brick

Recovery Shake (recipes start on page 223)

Dinner—3 bricks

Bacon-Wrapped Sea Scallops (page 206)

18 steamed asparagus spears

1 cup spaghetti squash

Water (no caffeine after 3:00 p.m.)

Snack—1 brick

1½ slices deli turkey, 1 tablespoon raisins, 18 peanuts

THE MAINTAINER MENUS FOR FRAME 2 (FORCE)

Remember that for each frame, you usually eat a range of bricks. Adjust up and down within that range for your own needs. Feel free to substitute any meal with a Meal Replacement Shake (recipes start on page 227).

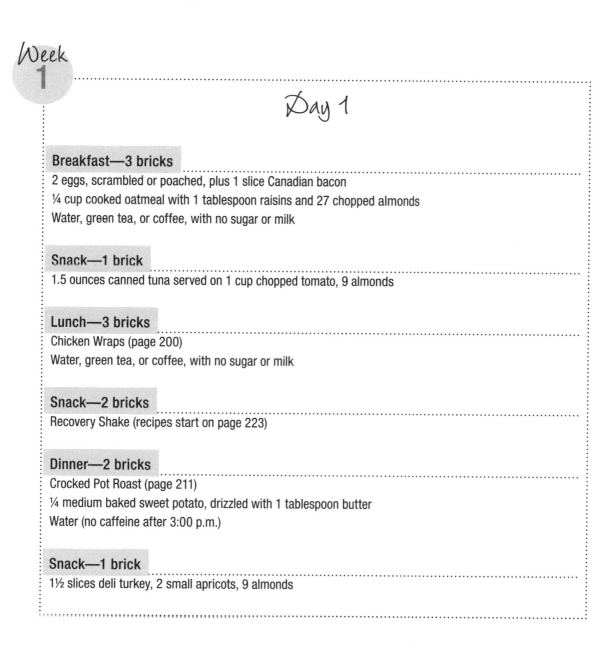

Week 1

Day 1

Breakfast—3 bricks
2 eggs, scrambled or poached, plus 1 slice Canadian bacon
¼ cup cooked oatmeal with 1 tablespoon raisins and 27 chopped almonds
Water, green tea, or coffee, with no sugar or milk

Snack—1 brick
1.5 ounces canned tuna served on 1 cup chopped tomato, 9 almonds

Lunch—3 bricks
Chicken Wraps (page 200)
Water, green tea, or coffee, with no sugar or milk

Snack—2 bricks
Recovery Shake (recipes start on page 223)

Dinner—2 bricks
Crocked Pot Roast (page 211)
¼ medium baked sweet potato, drizzled with 1 tablespoon butter
Water (no caffeine after 3:00 p.m.)

Snack—1 brick
1½ slices deli turkey, 2 small apricots, 9 almonds

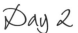

Day 2

Breakfast—3 bricks

3 eggs, scrambled
1 cup pineapple mixed with ¼ cup blueberries
4½ teaspoons of peanut butter
Water, green tea, or coffee, with no sugar or milk

Snack—1 brick

¼ cup cottage cheese mixed with 1 tablespoon raisins and 9 chopped almonds

Lunch—3 bricks

5 ounces canned tuna served over 2 cups mixed greens, ½ cup bean sprouts, and ¼ cup chopped onions and drizzled with 1 tablespoon balsamic vinegar
27 almonds
Water, green tea, or coffee, with no sugar or milk

Snack—2 bricks

Recovery Shake (recipes start on page 223)

Dinner—2 bricks

2 ounces pork chop, grilled or pan-fried
1 cup cooked Brussels sprouts
1 teaspoon olive oil on Brussels sprouts
6 teaspoons sour cream for pork chops
Water (no caffeine after 3:00 p.m.)

Snack—1 brick

1.5 ounces canned tuna served on 1 cup chopped tomato, 9 almonds

Day 3

Breakfast—3 bricks

Mini Quiche (page 195)

Water, green tea, or coffee, with no sugar or milk

Snack—1 brick

1.5 ounces ground turkey, ¼ apple with 1½ teaspoons peanut butter

Lunch—3 bricks

4.5 ounces cooked ground beef mixed with ⅓ cup tomato sauce and ¼ cup cooked onions and served over 1 cup spaghetti squash

27 almonds

Water, green tea, or coffee, with no sugar or milk

Snack—2 bricks

Recovery Shake (recipes start on page 223)

Dinner—3 bricks

3 ounces veal chop, covered with ⅓ cup tomato sauce

2 cups mixed raw greens, drizzled with 1 tablespoon balsamic vinegar

27 almonds

Water (no caffeine after 3:00 p.m.)

Snack—1 brick

1 hard-boiled egg, ¼ apple with 1½ teaspoons peanut butter

Day 4

Breakfast—3 bricks

2 eggs scrambled with 1 ounce chopped ham

¼ cup cranberries mixed with ⅓ cup grapefruit pieces

27 chopped almonds mixed in with berries

Water, green tea, or coffee, with no sugar or milk

Snack—1 brick

1½ slices deli ham, 1 cup red bell pepper slices, 9 almonds

Lunch—3 bricks

4.5 ounces ground turkey

1 cup cooked green beans, sprinkled with 27 crushed almonds

⅓ cup cooked carrots

Water, green tea, or coffee, with no sugar or milk

Snack—2 bricks

Recovery Shake (recipes start on page 223)

Dinner—2 bricks

3 ounces grilled chicken breast

1 cup spaghetti squash topped with ¼ cup tomato sauce mixed with ¼ cup cooked onion

18 almonds

Water (no caffeine after 3:00 p.m.)

Snack—1 brick

1.5 ounces grilled chicken breast, ¼ apple with 1½ teaspoons peanut butter

Day 5

Breakfast—3 bricks

6 egg whites, scrambled

1 kiwi with 1 plum

4½ teaspoons of almond butter

Water, green tea, or coffee, with no sugar or milk

Snack—1 brick each

1.5 ounces canned tuna served on ⅓ cup chopped tomato, 9 almonds

Lunch—3 bricks

Spinach Salad (page 201)

Water, green tea, or coffee, with no sugar or milk

Snack—2 bricks

Recovery Shake (recipes start on page 223)

Dinner—2 bricks

Shrimp Scampi (page 204)

2 cups cooked cabbage

Water (no caffeine after 3:00 p.m.)

Snack—1 brick

1.5 ounces grilled chicken breast, 2 or 3 celery sticks spread with 1½ teaspoons almond butter

Day 6

Breakfast—3 bricks

2 eggs scrambled with 1.5 ounces ground turkey

¼ cup oatmeal with 3 teaspoons peanut butter mixed in

⅓ cup blueberries

9 almonds shaved over blueberries

Water, green tea, or coffee, with no sugar or milk

Snack—1 brick

1.5 ounces grilled chicken breast, Zucchini Chips (½ cup) (page 222), 9 almonds

Lunch—3 bricks

Naked Taco Salad (page 201)

Water, green tea, or coffee, with no sugar or milk

Snack—2 bricks

Recovery Shake (recipes start on page 223)

Dinner—2 bricks

Low-Carb Lovers' Pizza (page 212)

18 almonds

Water (no caffeine after 3:00 p.m.)

Snack—1 brick

1½ slices deli ham, ½ cup red bell pepper slices, 15 olives

Day 7

Breakfast—3 bricks

6 egg whites scrambled with ½ cup cooked mushrooms

⅔ cup grapefruit sections

4½ teaspoons almond butter

Water, green tea, or coffee, with no sugar or milk

Snack—1 brick

Badass Eggs (2 halves) (page 220)

1¼ cups raw broccoli

Lunch—3 bricks

Sweet Tuna Salad (page 200)

Water, green tea, or coffee, with no sugar or milk

Snack—2 bricks

Recovery Shake (recipes start on page 223)

Dinner—3 bricks

3 ounces salmon with 2 teaspoons cocktail sauce

9 steamed asparagus spears

6 ounces baked sweet potato topped with 4 teaspoons peanut butter

Water (no caffeine after 3:00 p.m.)

Snack—1 brick

1½ slices deli turkey, 1 tablespoon raisins, 1½ teaspoons cashew butter

THE MAINTAINER MENUS FOR FRAME 3 (POWER)

Remember that in each frame, you usually eat a range of bricks. Adjust up and down within that range for your own needs. Feel free to substitute any meal with a Meal Replacement Shake (recipes start on page 227).

Week
1

Day 1

Breakfast—3 bricks
Mexican Omelet (page 194)
Water, green tea, or coffee, with no sugar or milk

Snack—1 brick
Recovery Shake (recipes start on page 223)

Lunch—3 bricks
4.5 ounces grilled chicken breast served over 1 cup lettuce and 1 cup chopped tomato and drizzled with
   1 tablespoon balsamic vinegar
1 plum
27 almonds
Water, green tea, or coffee, with no sugar or milk

Snack—2 bricks
3 ounces tuna on ⅓ cup chopped tomato and ½ chopped cucumber, 18 almonds

Dinner—3 bricks
3 ounces sirloin steak
9 steamed asparagus spears
½ small baked sweet potato, topped with 4 tablespoons cashew butter
Water, green tea, or coffee, with no sugar or milk

Snack—1 brick
1.5 ounces grilled chicken breast, 2 small apricots, 9 almonds

Day 2

Breakfast—3 bricks

3 eggs, scrambled

¾ apple

4½ teaspoons peanut butter

Water, green tea, or coffee, with no sugar or milk

Snack—1 brick

Recovery Shake (recipes start on page 223)

Lunch—3 bricks

4.5 ounces canned tuna served over 1½ cups chopped kale, ⅓ cup tomato

9 teaspoons sour cream mixed into tuna, kale, and tomato

Water, green tea, or coffee, with no sugar or milk

Snack—2 bricks

Recovery Shake (recipes start on page 223)

Dinner—3 bricks

Smothered Pork Chops (page 213)

1 cup sautéed cabbage

Water (no caffeine after 3:00 p.m.)

Snack—1 brick

1.5 ounces canned tuna served on 1 cup chopped tomato, 9 almonds

Day 3

Breakfast—3 bricks

Mini Quiche (page 195)

Water, green tea, or coffee, with no sugar or milk

Snack—1 brick

Recovery Shake (recipes start on page 223)

Lunch—3 bricks

4.5 ounces cooked ground beef mixed with ⅓ cup tomato sauce and ¼ cup cooked onion and served over
   1 cup spaghetti squash

27 almonds

Water, green tea, or coffee, with no sugar or milk

Snack—2 bricks

3 ounces grilled ground chicken, 6 ounces sweet potato, 3 teaspoons peanut butter all mashed together

Dinner—3 bricks

3 ounces veal chop

1½ cups kale, ⅓ cup chopped tomato drizzled with 1 tablespoon olive oil mixed with 6 teaspoons
   sour cream

Water (no caffeine after 3:00 p.m.)

Snack—1 brick

1 hard-boiled egg, ¼ apple with 1½ teaspoons peanut butter

Day 4

Breakfast—3 bricks

2 eggs scrambled with 1 ounce chopped ham

¾ orange

3 teaspoons peanut butter on eggs and ham

Water, green tea, or coffee

Snack—1 brick

Recovery Shake (recipes start on page 223)

Lunch—3 bricks

4.5 ounces ground turkey

1 cup cooked green beans, sprinkled with 27 crushed almonds

⅓ cup cooked carrots

Water, green tea, or coffee, with no sugar or milk

Snack—2 bricks

½ cup cottage cheese, 1 cup chopped fresh pineapple, 2¼ teaspoons sunflower seeds

Dinner—3 bricks

4.5 ounces grilled chicken breast

1 cup spaghetti squash topped with ⅓ cup tomato sauce mixed with ¼ cup cooked onion

27 almonds

Water (no caffeine after 3:00 p.m.)

Snack—1 brick

1½ slices turkey deli meat, ¼ apple with 1½ teaspoons peanut butter

Day 5

Breakfast—3 bricks

Grain-Free Granola with Badass Eggs (pages 196, 220)

Water, green tea, or coffee, with no sugar or milk

Snack—1 brick

Recovery Shake (recipes start on page 223)

Lunch—3 bricks

Spinach Salad (page 201)

Water, green tea, or coffee, with no sugar or milk

Snack—2 bricks

3 ounces canned tuna served on 2 cups chopped tomato, 18 almonds

Dinner—3 bricks

Blackened Whitefish (page 202)

Italian Salad (page 215)

6 teaspoons sour cream on salad

9 cashews chopped on whitefish

Water (no caffeine after 3:00 p.m.)

Snack—1 brick

1.5 ounces grilled chicken breast, 2 to 3 celery sticks spread with 1½ teaspoons peanut butter

Day 6

Breakfast—3 bricks

4.5 ounces ground turkey mixed with ¼ cup mashed butternut squash

½ slice of bread with 3 teaspoons cream cheese

6 teaspoons peanut butter on top turkey and butternut squash

Water, green tea, or coffee, with no sugar or milk

Snack—1 brick

Recovery Shake (recipes start on page 223)

Lunch—3 bricks

Naked Taco Salad (page 201)

Water, green tea, or coffee, with no sugar or milk

Snack—2 bricks

3 ounces grilled chicken breast, ½ cup red bell pepper slices, 3 teaspoons peanut butter

Dinner—3 bricks

3 ounces cooked ground beef mixed with ⅓ cup tomato sauce and ¼ cup onions served over
    1 cup spaghetti squash

27 almonds

Water (no caffeine after 3:00 p.m.)

Snack—1 brick

1½ slices deli turkey, ½ cup red bell pepper slices, 9 almonds

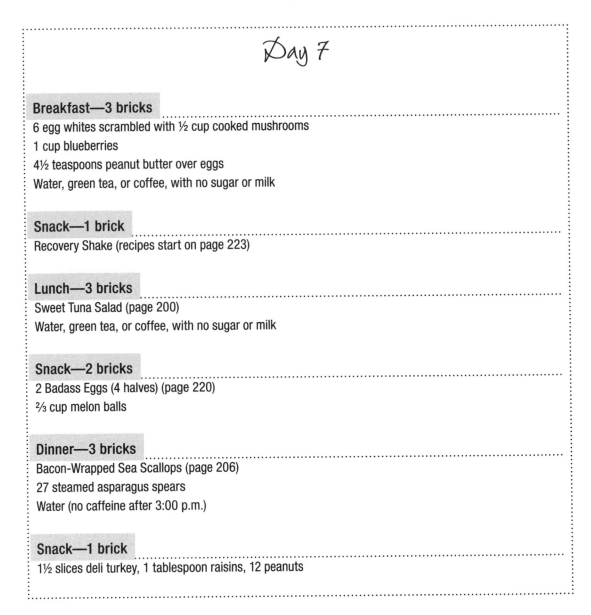

Day 7

Breakfast—3 bricks

6 egg whites scrambled with ½ cup cooked mushrooms

1 cup blueberries

4½ teaspoons peanut butter over eggs

Water, green tea, or coffee, with no sugar or milk

Snack—1 brick

Recovery Shake (recipes start on page 223)

Lunch—3 bricks

Sweet Tuna Salad (page 200)

Water, green tea, or coffee, with no sugar or milk

Snack—2 bricks

2 Badass Eggs (4 halves) (page 220)

⅔ cup melon balls

Dinner—3 bricks

Bacon-Wrapped Sea Scallops (page 206)

27 steamed asparagus spears

Water (no caffeine after 3:00 p.m.)

Snack—1 brick

1½ slices deli turkey, 1 tablespoon raisins, 12 peanuts

THE MAINTAINER MENUS FOR FRAME 4 (BOLD)

Remember that in each frame, you usually eat a range of bricks. Adjust up and down within that range for your own needs. Feel free to substitute any meal with a Meal Replacement Shake (recipes start on page 227).

Week 1

Day 1

Breakfast—3 bricks
Mini Quiche (page 195)
Water, green tea, or coffee, with no sugar or milk

Snack—2 bricks
Recovery Shake (recipes start on page 223)

Lunch—3 bricks
Chicken Vegetable Soup (page 197)
Water, green tea, or coffee, with no sugar or milk

Snack—2 bricks
3 ounces chopped baked or grilled chicken breast served on 2 cups chopped tomato, 18 almonds

Dinner—3 bricks
3 ounces sirloin steak
9 steamed asparagus spears
6 ounces baked sweet potato, topped with 2 tablespoons sour cream
Water (no caffeine after 3:00 p.m.)

Snack—1 brick
1 hard-boiled egg, 2 small apricots, 9 almonds

Day 2

Breakfast—3 bricks

3 eggs, scrambled

½ apple with 4½ teaspoons peanut butter

1 small plum

Water, green tea, or coffee, with no sugar or milk

Snack—2 bricks

Recovery Shake (recipes start on page 223)

Lunch—3 bricks

4.5 ounces canned tuna served over ¾ cup kale and ⅓ cup tomato and drizzled with 1 tablespoon
     balsamic vinegar

1½ teaspoons sunflower seeds mixed in with salad

27 almonds

Water, green tea, or coffee, with no sugar or milk

Snack—2 bricks

3 slices deli turkey, with 2 tablespoons of raisins and 18 chopped almonds

Dinner—3 bricks

3 ounces pork chop, grilled or pan-fried

1 cup cooked Brussels sprouts, prepared with 1 teaspoon olive oil

⅓ cup beets

18 almonds

Water (no caffeine after 3:00 p.m.)

Snack—1 brick

1.5 ounces canned tuna served on 1 cup chopped tomato, 9 almonds

Day 3

Breakfast—3 bricks
Mini Quiche (page 195)
Water, green tea, or coffee, with no sugar or milk

Snack—2 bricks
Recovery Shake (recipes start on page 223)

Lunch—3 bricks
Low-Carb Lovers' Pizza (page 212)
27 almonds
Water, green tea, or coffee, with no sugar or milk

Snack—2 bricks
3 ounces ground turkey, 1 cup Brussels sprouts with 1 tablespooon peanut butter

Dinner—3 bricks
3 ounces veal chop, covered with ⅓ cup tomato sauce
¾ cup kale and ⅓ cup chopped tomato drizzled with 1 tablespoon balsamic vinegar
27 almonds
Water (no caffeine after 3:00 p.m.)

Snack—1 brick
1 hard-boiled egg, ¼ apple with 1½ teaspoons peanut butter

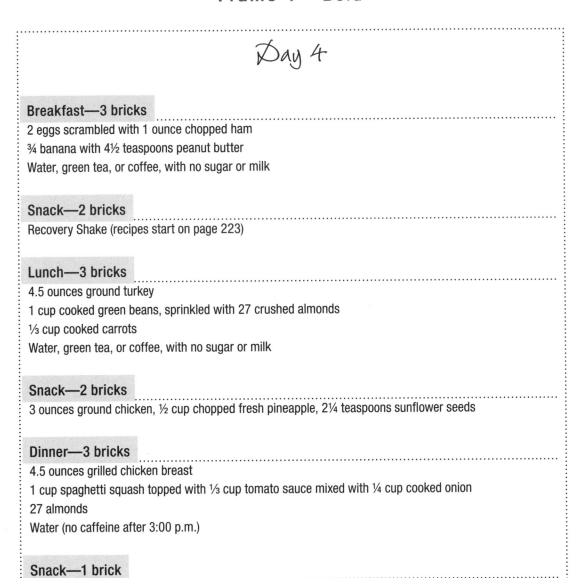

Day 4

Breakfast—3 bricks

2 eggs scrambled with 1 ounce chopped ham

¾ banana with 4½ teaspoons peanut butter

Water, green tea, or coffee, with no sugar or milk

Snack—2 bricks

Recovery Shake (recipes start on page 223)

Lunch—3 bricks

4.5 ounces ground turkey

1 cup cooked green beans, sprinkled with 27 crushed almonds

⅓ cup cooked carrots

Water, green tea, or coffee, with no sugar or milk

Snack—2 bricks

3 ounces ground chicken, ½ cup chopped fresh pineapple, 2¼ teaspoons sunflower seeds

Dinner—3 bricks

4.5 ounces grilled chicken breast

1 cup spaghetti squash topped with ⅓ cup tomato sauce mixed with ¼ cup cooked onion

27 almonds

Water (no caffeine after 3:00 p.m.)

Snack—1 brick

1 ounce pork, ¼ apple with 1½ teaspoons peanut butter

Day 5

Breakfast—3 bricks

3 eggs poached and served on top of 1 cup sautéed spinach

½ slice bread

27 almonds

Water, green tea, or coffee, with no sugar or milk

Snack—2 bricks

Recovery Shake (recipes start on page 223)

Lunch—3 bricks

Spinach Salad (page 201)

Water, green tea, or coffee, with no sugar or milk

Snack—1 brick

1.3 ounces canned tuna served on 1 cup chopped tomato, 9 almonds

Dinner—3 bricks

4.5 ounces catfish, baked or grilled, served with 2 tablespoons cocktail sauce

Creamy Coleslaw (page 216)

Water (no caffeine after 3:00 p.m.)

Snack—1 brick

1.5 ounces grilled chicken breast, 2 to 3 celery sticks spread with 1½ teaspoons peanut butter

Day 6

Breakfast—3 bricks

Grain-Free Granola and Badass Eggs (pages 196, 220)

Water, green tea, or coffee, with no sugar or milk

Snack—2 bricks

Recovery Shake (recipes start on page 223)

Lunch—3 bricks

Stuffed Tomato with Crab Salad (page 199)

Water, green tea, or coffee, with no sugar or milk

Snack—2 bricks

3 ounces grilled chicken breast, 1 cup red bell pepper slices, 6 teaspoons cream cheese

Dinner—3 bricks

"Spaghetti" and Meatballs (page 209)

Water (no caffeine after 3:00 p.m.)

Snack—1 brick

1 slice deli ham, ½ cup red bell pepper slices, 9 almonds

Day 7

Breakfast—3 bricks

6 egg whites, scrambled

¾ cup blueberries

4½ teaspoons peanut butter on top eggs

Water, green tea, or coffee, with no sugar or milk

Snack—2 bricks

Recovery Shake (recipes start on page 223)

Lunch—3 bricks

4.5 ounces canned tuna served on ¾ cup kale and ⅓ cup chopped tomato

27 almonds

⅓ cup raspberries

Water, green tea, or coffee, with no sugar or milk

Snack—2 bricks

2 Badass Eggs (4 halves) (page 220)

⅔ cup melon balls

Dinner—3 bricks

"Smoked" Salmon (page 203)

27 steamed asparagus spears, drizzled with 1 tablespoon of butter

Water (no caffeine after 3:00 p.m.)

Snack—1 brick

1½ slices deli turkey, 1 tablespoon raisins, 18 peanuts

THE MAINTAINER MENUS FOR FRAME 5 (CONFIDENT)

Remember that in each frame, you usually eat a range of bricks. Adjust up and down within that range for your own needs. Feel free to substitute any meal with a Meal Replacement Shake (recipes start on page 227).

Week 1

Day 1

Breakfast—3 bricks

2 eggs, scrambled or poached, with 1 slice Canadian bacon

½ apple with 4½ teaspoons peanut butter

1 small plum

Water, green tea, or coffee, with no sugar or milk

Snack—3 bricks

4.5 ounces canned tuna served on 1½ cups chopped kale, ⅓ cup chopped tomato, 27 almonds

Lunch—4 bricks

Chicken Wraps (page 200)

Water, green tea, or coffee, with no sugar or milk

Snack—2 bricks

Recovery Shake (recipes start on page 223)

Dinner—3 bricks

4 ounces sirloin steak

9 steamed asparagus spears

½ cup cooked Brussels sprouts, drizzled with 1 tablespoon of butter

⅓ cup beets

Water (no caffeine after 3:00 p.m.)

Snack—1 brick

1.5 ounces ground turkey, 2 small apricots, 9 almonds

Day 2

Breakfast—3 bricks

3 eggs, scrambled

¾ apple

4½ teaspoons almond butter

Water, green tea, or coffee, with no sugar or milk

Snack—3 bricks

1½ cups cottage cheese, mixed with 3 tablespoons raisins and 27 chopped almonds

Lunch—4 bricks

5 ounces canned tuna served over 1½ cups kale, ⅓ cup beets, ¼ cup butternut squash cubed and
    drizzled with 1 tablespoon balsamic vinegar

27 almonds

Water, green tea, or coffee, with no sugar or milk

Snack—2 bricks

Recovery Shake (recipes start on page 223)

Dinner—3 bricks

3 ounces pork chop, grilled or pan-fried

1 cup cooked Brussels sprouts, drizzled with 1 tablespoon of olive oil

½ cup cooked okra

6 tablespoons sour cream on pork chops

Water (no caffeine after 3:00 p.m.)

Snack—1 brick

1.5 ounces canned tuna served on 1 cup chopped tomato, 9 almonds

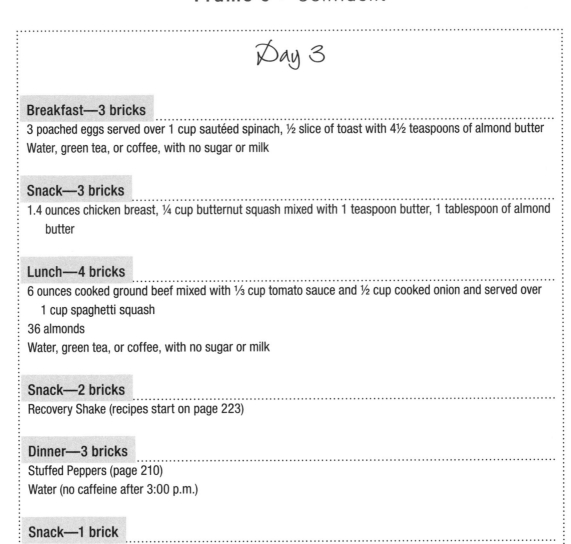

Day 3

Breakfast—3 bricks

3 poached eggs served over 1 cup sautéed spinach, ½ slice of toast with 4½ teaspoons of almond butter

Water, green tea, or coffee, with no sugar or milk

Snack—3 bricks

1.4 ounces chicken breast, ¼ cup butternut squash mixed with 1 teaspoon butter, 1 tablespoon of almond butter

Lunch—4 bricks

6 ounces cooked ground beef mixed with ⅓ cup tomato sauce and ½ cup cooked onion and served over 1 cup spaghetti squash

36 almonds

Water, green tea, or coffee, with no sugar or milk

Snack—2 bricks

Recovery Shake (recipes start on page 223)

Dinner—3 bricks

Stuffed Peppers (page 210)

Water (no caffeine after 3:00 p.m.)

Snack—1 brick

Egg Muffin Snacks (page 221)

Day 4

Breakfast—3 bricks

2 eggs scrambled with 1 ounce ham (cubed)

½ cup pineapple mixed with 5 cherries

4½ teaspoons cashew butter

Water, green tea, or coffee, with no sugar or milk

Snack—3 bricks

1½ ounces grilled salmon mixed with 1 cup chopped fresh pineapple and ½ kiwi topped with
2¼ teaspoons sunflower seeds

Lunch—4 bricks

6 ounces ground turkey

1½ cups sautéed kale mixed with ½ cup sautéed leeks, ⅓ cup chopped tomato, and 1 teaspoon olive oil

36 almonds

Water, green tea, or coffee, with no sugar or milk

Snack—2 bricks

Recovery Shake (recipes start on page 223)

Dinner—3 bricks

5 ounces grilled chicken breast

1 cup spaghetti squash topped with ⅓ cup tomato sauce mixed with ¼ cup cooked onion topped with
9 teaspoons sour cream

Water (no caffeine after 3:00 p.m.)

Snack—1 brick

1.5 ounces ground turkey, ¼ apple with 1½ teaspoons peanut butter

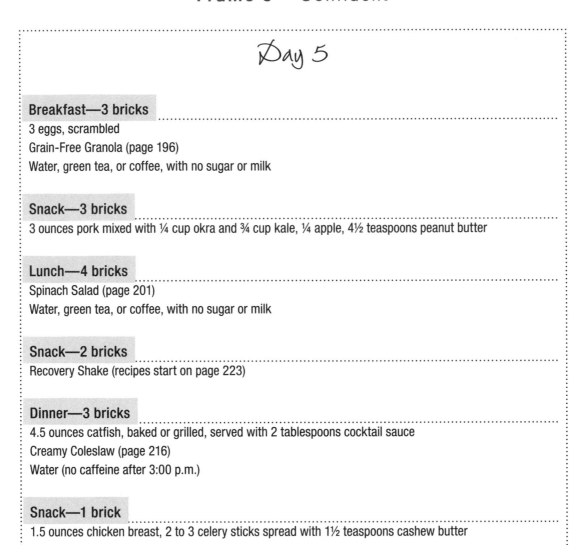

Day 5

Breakfast—3 bricks

3 eggs, scrambled

Grain-Free Granola (page 196)

Water, green tea, or coffee, with no sugar or milk

Snack—3 bricks

3 ounces pork mixed with ¼ cup okra and ¾ cup kale, ¼ apple, 4½ teaspoons peanut butter

Lunch—4 bricks

Spinach Salad (page 201)

Water, green tea, or coffee, with no sugar or milk

Snack—2 bricks

Recovery Shake (recipes start on page 223)

Dinner—3 bricks

4.5 ounces catfish, baked or grilled, served with 2 tablespoons cocktail sauce

Creamy Coleslaw (page 216)

Water (no caffeine after 3:00 p.m.)

Snack—1 brick

1.5 ounces chicken breast, 2 to 3 celery sticks spread with 1½ teaspoons cashew butter

Day 6

Breakfast—3 bricks

3 ounces turkey sausage

15 cherries

4½ teaspoons cashew butter

Water, green tea, or coffee, with no sugar or milk

Snack—3 bricks

4.5 ounces grilled chicken breast, 1½ cups red bell pepper slices, 9 teaspoons cream cheese

Lunch—4 bricks

Naked Taco Salad (page 201)

Water, green tea, or coffee, with no sugar or milk

Snack—2 bricks

Recovery Shake (recipes start on page 223)

Dinner—3 bricks

4.5 ounces cooked ground turkey mixed with ⅓ cup tomato sauce

1 cup sautéed spinach

½ cup okra

27 almonds

Water (no caffeine after 3:00 p.m.)

Snack—1 brick

1 slice deli ham, ½ cup red bell pepper slices, 9 almonds

Day 7

Breakfast—3 bricks

6 egg whites scrambled with ½ cup cooked mushrooms

9 ounces baked sweet potato

4½ teaspoons peanut butter

Water, green tea, or coffee, with no sugar or milk

Snack—3 bricks

3 Badass Eggs (6 halves) (page 220)

Lunch—4 bricks

Sweet Tuna Salad (page 200)

Water, green tea, or coffee, with no sugar or milk

Snack—2 bricks

Recovery Shake (recipes start on page 223)

Dinner—3 bricks

4.5 ounces salmon with 1 tablespoon cocktail sauce

Sautéed Greens (page 217)

1 cup spaghetti squash

4½ teaspoons sour cream

Water (no caffeine after 3:00 p.m.)

Snack—1 brick

1 slice deli turkey, 1 tablespoon raisins, 9 peanuts

I'M A BADASS

Barbara, age 46, and her husband attended one of my seminars. Afterward, they started the program. Barbara lost nearly 15 pounds in 21 days by following the Modifier plan.

She "graduated" to the Maintainer plan, and her weight continued to fall off. At the same time, she followed my workout plan to get her butt in shape.

Barbara wrote me: "I was completely blown away by how simple your food plan is—and how easy it is to stay on and not feel deprived. My husband lost weight, too, and it was great having him on board with me. It really lifted our spirits to do something together that was not only good for us physically but brought us together emotionally. We're still going through the plan. It continues to be easy to implement on a daily basis."

CHAPTER 9

The Badass Meal Plans for Gainers

PACKING ON SEXY LEAN muscle quickly means getting critical amounts of the three macros in your body throughout the day. These meal plans will help you do just that. I've broken it all down for you, nice and simple. All you have to do is work out hard, eat well, and track your beautifully developing body in the mirror.

One of the keys on the Gainer plan is meal timing. You've got to be strict here. The critical window of opportunity for building gorgeous muscle is around your workout. That's the part of the day when you want to pack your body with protein and carbs to grow muscle. In addition to my post-workout Recovery Shakes, I also advise sipping a shake during your workout to gain even more muscle.

Okay, let's get into the specifics.

THE 6 PRINCIPLES OF CHRISTMAS FOR GAINERS

I have 6 simple principles to help you get the best results. If you're unsure of anything, refer to these guidelines.

1. Do not start the Gainer plan unless you have completed the Maintainer plan for 21 strict days.

2. Follow the plan strictly for 21 days, observing how many bricks you eat at meals. You don't have to clean your plate. When you feel full, stop eating.

3. Choose primo and acceptable foods with booty foods when planning your meals. You have the most flexibility on food quality in this category. Refer to my chart Hip Advice: Booty Foods at a Glance on page 47 for a list of booty foods. Feel free to replace any meal or snack with a Meal Replacement Shake (recipes start on page 227).

4. Have your breakfast within 45 minutes after waking up. This is imperative to jump-start your metabolism. Do not go more than five daytime hours without eating.

5. Have a Recovery Shake daily on this plan, one immediately within minutes of completing your workout, before your cool-down starts! See my Recovery Shake recipes for ideas; they begin on page 223. This recovery shake does not count toward your daily brick intake. You can also have up to two meal replacement shakes on this plan.

6. Drink 8 to 10 cups (64–80 ounces) of pure water daily, in addition to coffee and green tea. Do not drink any sodas or other naturally or artificially sweetened beverages. No diet soda!

THE GAINER MENUS FOR FRAME 1 (MIGHTY)

Remember that for each frame, you are permitted to eat within a range of bricks (see page 63). Adjust up and down within that range for your own needs. Feel free to substitute any meal with a Meal Replacement Shake (recipes start on page 227).

Day 1

Breakfast—2 bricks

1 egg, scrambled or poached; 1 slice Canadian bacon

½ cup blueberries

3 teaspoons peanut butter

Water, green tea, or coffee, with no sugar or milk

Snack—1 brick

1.5 ounces canned tuna mixed with 3 tablespoons avocado and served on 1 cup chopped tomato

Lunch—3 bricks

Chicken Wraps (page 200)

6 ounces sweet potato

9 tablespoons avocado

Water, green tea, or coffee with no sugar or milk

Snack—2 bricks

Recovery Shake (recipes start on page 223)

Dinner—3 bricks

4.5 ounces tuna steak

18 steamed asparagus spears

1 cup sautéed spinach

9 teaspoons sour cream

Water (no caffeine after 3:00 p.m.)

Snack—1 brick

Recovery Shake (recipes start on page 223)

Day 2

Breakfast—2 bricks

Mexican Omelet (page 194)

Water, green tea, or coffee, with no sugar or milk

Snack—1 brick

¼ cup cottage cheese, mixed with 1 tablespoon raisins and 9 chopped almonds

Lunch—3 bricks

4.5 ounces canned tuna served over 1½ cups sautéed kale and ⅓ cup chopped tomato and 9 teaspoons
    sour cream on top

Water, green tea, or coffee, with no sugar or milk

Snack—2 bricks

Recovery Shake (recipes start on page 223)

Dinner—3 bricks

Smothered Pork Chops (page 213)

½ cup cooked quinoa

Water (no caffeine after 3:00 p.m.)

Snack—1 brick

Recovery Shake (recipes start on page 223)

Day 3

Breakfast—2 bricks
2 poached eggs

½ orange

3 teaspoons almond butter

Water, green tea, or coffee, with no sugar or milk

Snack—1 brick
3 ounces ground pork, ¼ apple with 1½ teaspoons peanut butter

Lunch—3 bricks
4.5 ounces cooked ground beef mixed with ⅓ cup tomato sauce and ⅓ cup chopped tomatoes and served
over ¼ cup quinoa with 9 tablespoons chopped avocado mixed in

Water, green tea, or coffee, with no sugar or milk

Snack—2 bricks
Recovery Shake (recipes start on page 223)

Dinner—3 bricks
Shrimp Scampi (page 204) with 6 teaspoons cream cheese mixed in

2 cups mixed raw greens

½ cup mashed butternut squash with 1 teaspoon butter

Water (no caffeine after 3:00 p.m.)

Snack—1 brick
Recovery Shake (recipes start on page 223)

Day 4

Breakfast—2 bricks
Mini Quiche (page 195)
Water, green tea, or coffee, with no sugar or milk

Snack—1 brick
1 slice deli ham, ½ cup red bell pepper slices, 9 almonds

Lunch—3 bricks
4.5 ounces ground turkey
½ cup cooked green beans, sprinkled with 18 crushed almonds and drizzled with 1 teaspoon butter
⅔ cup cooked carrots
Water, green tea, or coffee, with no sugar or milk

Snack—2 bricks
Recovery Shake (recipes start on page 223)

Dinner—3 bricks
4.5 ounces grilled chicken breast
½ cup spaghetti squash topped with ⅓ cup tomato sauce mixed with ¼ cup cooked onion
½ avocado, drizzled with 1 teaspoon olive oil
Water (no caffeine after 3:00 p.m.)

Snack—1 brick
Recovery Shake (recipes start on page 223)

Day 5

Breakfast—2 bricks

4 egg whites, scrambled

¼ cup oatmeal cooked with 1 tablespoon raisins, and 6 tablespoons half-and-half

Water, green tea, or coffee, with no sugar or milk

Snack—1 brick

1.5 ounces canned tuna mixed with 3 tablespoons avocado and served on ⅓ cup chopped tomato

Lunch—3 bricks

Spinach Salad (page 201)

Water, green tea, or coffee, with no sugar or milk

Snack—2 bricks

Recovery Shake (recipes start on page 223)

Dinner—3 bricks

4.5 ounces catfish, baked or grilled, served with 1 tablespoon cocktail sauce

Sautéed Greens (page 217)

⅓ cup cooked corn

4½ teaspoons sour cream on greens and fish

Water (no caffeine after 3:00 p.m.)

Snack—1 brick

Recovery Shake (recipes start on page 223)

Day 6

Breakfast—2 bricks

2 ounces turkey sausage

½ slice toast with 1 teaspoons butter

3 teaspoons peanut butter

Water, green tea, or coffee, with no sugar or milk

Snack—1 brick

1.5 ounces grilled chicken breast, ½ cup red bell pepper slices, 9 almonds

Lunch—3 bricks

Naked Taco Salad (page 201)

Water, green tea, or coffee, with no sugar or milk

Snack—2 bricks

Recovery Shake (recipes start on page 223)

Dinner—3 bricks

Low-Carb Lovers' Pizza (page 212)

27 almonds

Water (no caffeine after 3:00 p.m.)

Snack—1 brick

Recovery Shake (recipes start on page 223)

Day 7

Breakfast—2 bricks

4 egg whites, scrambled

1 slice bacon

½ piece toast

1½ teaspoons almond butter

Water, green tea, or coffee, with no sugar or milk

Snack—1 brick

Badass Eggs (2 halves) (page 220)

Lunch—3 bricks

4.5 ounces canned tuna mixed with 9 tablespoons mashed avocado, served over ½ cup quinoa and ⅓ cup chopped tomato

Water, green tea, or coffee, with no sugar or milk

Snack—2 bricks

Recovery Shake (recipes start on page 223)

Dinner—3 bricks

4.5 ounces salmon with 1 tablespoon cocktail sauce

9 steamed asparagus spears, drizzled with 1 tablespoon butter

6 ounces baked sweet potato

6 teaspoons sour cream

Water (no caffeine after 3:00 p.m.)

Snack—1 brick

Recovery Shake (recipes start on page 223)

THE GAINER MENUS FOR FRAME 2 (FORCE)

Remember that for each frame, you are permitted to eat within a range of bricks (see page 63). Adjust up and down within that range for your own needs. Feel free to substitute any meal with a Meal Replacement Shake (recipes start on page 227).

Week
1

Day 1

Breakfast—3 bricks
Mexican Omelet (page 194)
Water, green tea, or coffee, with no sugar or milk

Snack—1 brick
1.5 ounces canned tuna mixed with 3 tablespoons avocado served on 1 cup chopped tomato

Lunch—3 bricks
Chicken Vegetable Soup (page 197)
Water, green tea, or coffee, with no sugar or milk

Snack—2 bricks
Recovery Shake (recipes start on page 223)

Dinner—3 bricks
3 ounces sirloin steak topped with 1 teaspoon butter
18 steamed asparagus spears with 1 teaspoon butter
6 ounces baked sweet potato, topped with 3 tablespoons sour cream
Water (no caffeine after 3:00 p.m.)

Snack—1 brick
Recovery Shake (recipes start on page 223)

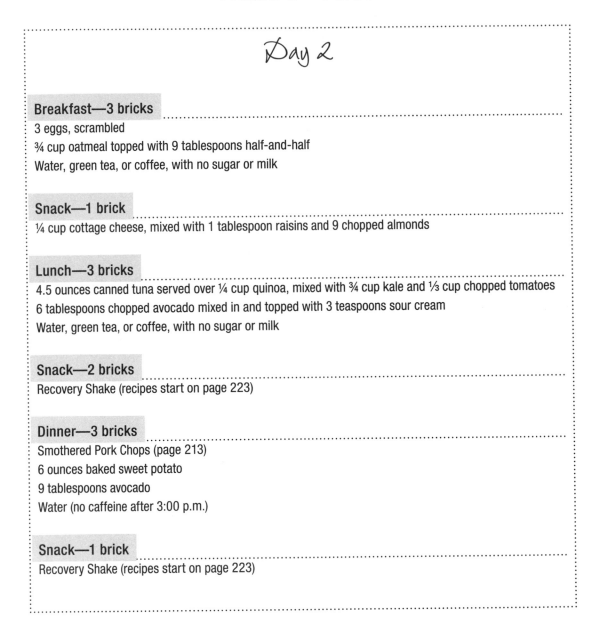

Day 2

Breakfast—3 bricks

3 eggs, scrambled

¾ cup oatmeal topped with 9 tablespoons half-and-half

Water, green tea, or coffee, with no sugar or milk

Snack—1 brick

¼ cup cottage cheese, mixed with 1 tablespoon raisins and 9 chopped almonds

Lunch—3 bricks

4.5 ounces canned tuna served over ¼ cup quinoa, mixed with ¾ cup kale and ⅓ cup chopped tomatoes

6 tablespoons chopped avocado mixed in and topped with 3 teaspoons sour cream

Water, green tea, or coffee, with no sugar or milk

Snack—2 bricks

Recovery Shake (recipes start on page 223)

Dinner—3 bricks

Smothered Pork Chops (page 213)

6 ounces baked sweet potato

9 tablespoons avocado

Water (no caffeine after 3:00 p.m.)

Snack—1 brick

Recovery Shake (recipes start on page 223)

Day 3

Breakfast—3 bricks

2 eggs scrambled with 1 slice Canadian bacon

½ slice of toast with 1 teaspoon butter

½ cup oatmeal served with 6 tablespoons half-and-half

Water, green tea, or coffee, with no sugar or milk

Snack—1 brick

¼ cup cottage cheese, ¼ apple with 1½ teaspoons peanut butter

Lunch—3 bricks

4.5 ounces cooked ground beef mixed with ⅓ cup tomato sauce and served over ½ cup cooked quinoa
    mixed with 6 tablespoons avocado and 3 teaspoons sour cream

Water, green tea, or coffee, with no sugar or milk

Snack—2 bricks

Recovery Shake (recipes start on page 223)

Dinner—3 bricks

3 ounces veal chop, covered with ½ cup tomato sauce

¾ cup kale drizzled with 1 tablespoon balsamic vinegar

4½ teaspoons almond butter

Water (no caffeine after 3:00 p.m.)

Snack—1 brick

Recovery Shake (recipes start on page 223)

Day 4

Breakfast—3 bricks

2 eggs scrambled with 1 ounce cubed ham

½ cup oatmeal cooked with 1 tablespoon raisins and topped with 9 tablespoons half-and-half

Water, green tea, or coffee, with no sugar or milk

Snack—1 brick

1 slice deli ham, 1 cup red bell pepper slices, 9 almonds

Lunch—3 bricks

4.5 ounces ground turkey

½ cup cooked white rice

3 tablespoons sour cream

6 tablespoons avocado

Water, green tea, or coffee, with no sugar or milk

Snack—2 bricks

Recovery Shake (recipes start on page 223)

Dinner—3 bricks

4.5 ounces grilled chicken breast

2 cups steamed broccoli

6 ounces baked sweet potato

¼ avocado

Water (no caffeine after 3:00 p.m.)

Snack—1 brick

Recovery Shake (recipes start on page 223)

Day 5

Breakfast—3 bricks

6 egg whites, scrambled

½ cup cooked oatmeal, served with 9 tablespoons half-and-half

Water, green tea, or coffee, with no sugar or milk

Snack—1 brick

1.5 ounces canned tuna mixed with 1 teaspoon mayonnaise and served on 1 cup chopped tomato

Lunch—3 bricks

Spinach Salad (page 201)

Water, green tea, or coffee, with no sugar or milk

Snack—2 bricks

Recovery Shake (recipes start on page 223)

Dinner—3 bricks

4.5 ounces catfish, baked or grilled, served with 1 tablespoon cocktail sauce

Creamy Coleslaw (page 216)

Water (no caffeine after 3:00 p.m.)

Snack—1 brick

Recovery Shake (recipes start on page 223)

Day 6

Breakfast—3 bricks
3 ounces turkey sausage

¾ bran muffin with 1 teaspoon butter and 3 teaspoons cream cheese

Water, green tea, or coffee, with no sugar or milk

Snack—1 brick
1.5 ounces grilled chicken breast, ½ cup red bell pepper slices, 1½ teaspoons cashew butter

Lunch—3 bricks
Naked Taco Salad (page 201)

Water, green tea, or coffee, with no sugar or milk

Snack—2 bricks
Recovery Shake (recipes start on page 223)

Dinner—3 bricks
Crocked Pot Roast (page 211)

18 almonds

Water (no caffeine after 3:00 p.m.)

Snack—1 brick
Recovery Shake (recipes start on page 223)

Day 7

Breakfast—3 bricks

6 egg whites scrambled with ¾ cup quinoa, ¾ cup chopped tomato with 9 tablespoons avocado mixed in
Water, green tea, or coffee, with no sugar or milk

Snack—1 brick

Badass Eggs (2 halves) (page 220)

Lunch—3 bricks

3 ounces canned tuna mixed with 9 tablespoons mashed avocado, served over ¾ cup kale and
⅓ cup chopped tomatoes
½ cup pineapple
⅓ cup raspberries
Water, green tea, or coffee, with no sugar or milk

Snack—2 bricks

Recovery Shake (recipes start on page 223)

Dinner—3 bricks

Coconut Shrimp (page 205)
9 steamed asparagus spears
6 ounces baked sweet potato
Water (no caffeine after 3:00 p.m.)

Snack—1 brick

Recovery Shake (recipes start on page 223)

THE GAINER MENUS FOR FRAME 3 (POWER)

Remember that for each frame, you are permitted to eat within a range of bricks (see page 63). Adjust up and down within that range for your own needs. Feel free to substitute any meal with a Meal Replacement Shake (recipes start on page 227).

Week 1

Day 1

Breakfast—3 bricks
2 eggs, scrambled or poached, with 1 slice Canadian bacon
¾ cup oatmeal cooked with 9 tablespoons half-and-half
Water, green tea, or coffee, with no sugar or milk

Snack—2 bricks
Recovery Shake (recipes start on page 223)

Lunch—4 bricks
Chicken Wraps (page 200)
6 ounces baked sweet potato
Water, green tea, or coffee, with no sugar or milk

Snack—2 bricks
3 ounces chopped baked or grilled chicken breast mixed with 2 teaspoons olive oil and served over 2 cups chopped tomato

Dinner—3 bricks
3 ounces sirloin steak
9 ounces sweet potato, topped with 1 teaspoon butter, 3 tablespoons sour cream, and 7½ teaspoons bacon bits
Water (no caffeine after 3:00 p.m.)

Snack—1 brick
Recovery Shake (recipes start on page 223)

Day 2

Breakfast—3 bricks

3 eggs, scrambled

½ cup pineapple mixed with 5 cherries

4½ teaspoons cashew butter on eggs

Water, green tea, or coffee, with no sugar or milk

Snack—2 bricks

Recovery Shake (recipes start on page 223)

Lunch—4 bricks

4.5 ounces canned tuna served over ¾ cup kale and ½ cup pineapple, and 1 tablespoon balsamic vinegar
    with 36 crushed cashews mixed in

Water, green tea, or coffee, with no sugar or milk

Snack—2 bricks

½ cup cottage cheese, mixed with 2 tablespoons raisins and 3 teaspoons peanut butter

Dinner—3 bricks

3 ounces pork chop, grilled or pan-fried

1 cup cooked Brussels sprouts, drizzled with 1 tablespoon butter

6 ounces baked sweet potato

3 teaspoons peanut butter

Water (no caffeine after 3:00 p.m.)

Snack—1 brick

Recovery Shake (recipes start on page 223)

Day 3

Breakfast—3 bricks

3 slices Canadian bacon, pan-fried

½ cup cooked grits with 3 teaspoons butter

Water, green tea, or coffee, with no sugar or milk

Snack—2 bricks

Recovery Shake (recipes start on page 223)

Lunch—4 bricks

6 ounces cooked ground beef mixed with ⅓ cup tomato sauce and ¼ cup cooked onion and served over
   ½ cup quinoa, 9 tablespoons avocado, and 3 tablespoons sour cream

Water, green tea, or coffee, with no sugar or milk

Snack—2 bricks

2 ounces beef, ½ apple, 3 teaspoons peanut butter

Dinner—3 bricks

Herb-Roasted Lamb (page 214)

¾ cup kale, drizzled with 1 tablespoon balsamic vinegar and 3 tablespoon avocado

6 ounces baked sweet potato topped with 1 teaspoon butter and 3 teaspoons sour cream

Water (no caffeine after 3:00 p.m.)

Snack—1 brick

Recovery Shake (recipes start on page 223)

Day 4

Breakfast—3 bricks

2 eggs scrambled with 1 ounce cubed ham

¾ cup oatmeal cooked with 4½ teaspoons peanut butter

Water, green tea, or coffee, with no sugar or milk

Snack—2 bricks

Recovery Shake (recipes start on page 223)

Lunch—4 bricks

6 ounces ground turkey

½ cup cooked green beans mixed with ¼ cup quinoa and sprinkled with 18 crushed almonds and drizzled
with 2 teaspoons melted butter

⅓ cup cooked carrots

Water, green tea, or coffee, with no sugar or milk

Snack—2 bricks

½ cup cottage cheese, ½ cup chopped fresh pineapple, 2¼ teaspoons sunflower seeds

Dinner—3 bricks

4.5 ounces grilled chicken breast

¾ cup kale sautéed with ⅓ cup tomato sauce mixed with ¼ cup cooked onion

¼ avocado, drizzled with 1 teaspoon butter

Water (no caffeine after 3:00 p.m.)

Snack—1 brick

Recovery Shake (recipes start on page 223)

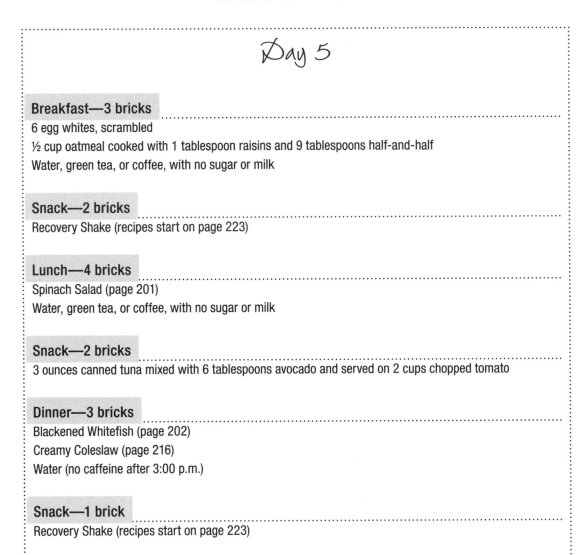

Day 5

Breakfast—3 bricks

6 egg whites, scrambled

½ cup oatmeal cooked with 1 tablespoon raisins and 9 tablespoons half-and-half

Water, green tea, or coffee, with no sugar or milk

Snack—2 bricks

Recovery Shake (recipes start on page 223)

Lunch—4 bricks

Spinach Salad (page 201)

Water, green tea, or coffee, with no sugar or milk

Snack—2 bricks

3 ounces canned tuna mixed with 6 tablespoons avocado and served on 2 cups chopped tomato

Dinner—3 bricks

Blackened Whitefish (page 202)

Creamy Coleslaw (page 216)

Water (no caffeine after 3:00 p.m.)

Snack—1 brick

Recovery Shake (recipes start on page 223)

Day 6

Breakfast—3 bricks

3 ounces turkey sausage

¾ bran muffin with 2 teaspoons butter

9 almonds

Water, green tea, or coffee, with no sugar or milk

Snack—2 bricks

Recovery Shake (recipes start on page 223)

Lunch—4 bricks

Naked Taco Salad (page 201)

Water, green tea, or coffee, with no sugar or milk

Snack—2 bricks

3 ounces grilled chicken breast, 1 cup red bell pepper slices, 6 teaspoons cream cheese

Dinner—3 bricks

4.5 ounces cooked ground beef mixed with ¾ cup kale sautéed with ⅓ cup tomato sauce and
1 tablespoon raisins with 9 tablespoons avocado chunks mixed in and topped with 3 teaspoons
sour cream

Water (no caffeine after 3:00 p.m.)

Snack—1 brick

Recovery Shake (recipes start on page 223)

Day 7

Breakfast—3 bricks

6 egg whites, scrambled

9 ounces mashed sweet potato in 1 teaspoon butter

3 teaspoons peanut butter

Water, green tea, or coffee, with no sugar or milk

Snack—2 bricks

Recovery Shake (recipes start on page 223)

Lunch—4 bricks

6 ounces canned tuna mixed with 12 tablespoons guacamole served over 2 cups chopped tomato

6 ounces baked sweet potato

Water, green tea, or coffee, with no sugar or milk

Snack—2 bricks

2 Badass Eggs (4 halves) (page 220)

Dinner—3 bricks

4.5 ounces salmon with 1 tablespoon cocktail sauce

1½ cups kale mixed with ⅓ cup cooked carrots, 6 tablespoons avocado, and 9 crushed cashews

Water (no caffeine after 3:00 p.m.)

Snack—1 brick

Recovery Shake (recipes start on page 223)

THE GAINER MENUS FOR FRAME 4 (BOLD)

Week **1**

Day 1

Breakfast—3 bricks

2 eggs, scrambled or poached, with 1 slice Canadian bacon

½ cup oatmeal cooked with 1 tablespoon raisins and 9 tablespoons half-and-half

Water, green tea, or coffee, with no sugar or milk

Snack—2 bricks

Recovery Shake (recipes start on page 223)

Lunch—3 bricks

4.5 ounces grilled chicken breast served over ¾ cup Swiss chard and ⅓ cup chopped tomato mixed with 1 tablespoon balsamic vinegar, 6 tablespoons chopped avocado, and 3 tablespoons sour cream

Water, green tea, or coffee, with no sugar or milk

Snack—2 bricks

3 ounces chopped baked or grilled chicken breast mixed with 2 teaspoons olive oil and served on ⅔ cup chopped tomato

Dinner—3 bricks

3 ounces sirloin steak

9 steamed asparagus spears

9 ounces baked sweet potato, topped with 1 teaspoon butter, 3 tablespoons sour cream, and 7½ teaspoons bacon bits

Water (no caffeine after 3:00 p.m.)

Snack—2 bricks

Recovery Shake (recipes start on page 223)

Day 2

Breakfast—3 bricks

3 eggs, scrambled

¾ cup oatmeal with 9 tablespoons half-and-half

Water, green tea, or coffee, with no sugar or milk

Snack—2 bricks

Recovery Shake (recipes start on page 223)

Lunch—3 bricks

4.5 ounces canned tuna served over ¾ cup kale and ½ cup pineapple with 9 tablespoons chopped avocado mixed in

Water, green tea, or coffee, with no sugar or milk

Snack—2 bricks

½ cup cottage cheese, mixed with 2 tablespoons raisins and 18 chopped almonds

Dinner—3 bricks

Smothered Pork Chops (page 213)

Water (no caffeine after 3:00 p.m.)

Snack—2 bricks

Recovery Shake (recipes start on page 223)

Day 3

Breakfast—3 bricks

Mexican Omelet (page 194)

Water, green tea, or coffee, with no sugar or milk

Snack—2 bricks

Recovery Shake (recipes start on page 223)

Lunch—3 bricks

4.5 ounces cooked ground beef mixed with ⅓ cup tomato sauce and served over ½ cup cooked pasta
   topped with 6 tablespoons avocado and 3 tablespoons sour cream

Water, green tea, or coffee, with no sugar or milk

Snack—2 bricks

½ cup cottage cheese, ½ cup shredded pineapple, 3 teaspoons peanut butter

Dinner—3 bricks

3 ounces veal chop

9 ounces baked sweet potato with 2 teaspoons butter and 3 tablespoons sour cream

Water (no caffeine after 3:00 p.m.)

Snack—2 bricks

Recovery Shake (recipes start on page 223)

Day 4

Breakfast—3 bricks

2 eggs scrambled with 1 ounce cubed ham

¾ cup cooked oatmeal mixed with 4½ teaspoons peanut butter

Water, green tea, or coffee, with no sugar or milk

Snack—2 bricks

Recovery Shake (recipes start on page 223)

Lunch—3 bricks

4.5 ounces ground turkey mashed in with 9 tablespoons avocado

¼ cup quinoa with ¾ cup cooked carrots

Water, green tea, or coffee, with no sugar or milk

Snack—2 bricks

½ cup cottage cheese, ½ cup chopped fresh pineapple, 2¼ teaspoons sunflower seeds

Dinner—3 bricks

4.5 ounces grilled chicken breast

⅓ cup tomato sauce served over ½ cup of quinoa

½ avocado

Water (no caffeine after 3:00 p.m.)

Snack—2 bricks

Recovery Shake (recipes start on page 223)

Day 5

Breakfast—3 bricks

6 egg whites, scrambled in 1½ teaspoons butter

½ cup oatmeal cooked with 1 tablespoon raisins and 6 tablespoons half-and-half

Water, green tea, or coffee, with no sugar or milk

Snack—2 bricks

Recovery Shake (recipes start on page 223)

Lunch—3 bricks

Spinach Salad (page 201)

Water, green tea, or coffee, with no sugar or milk

Snack—2 bricks

3 ounces canned tuna mixed with 2 teaspoons olive oil and served on 2 cups chopped tomato

Dinner—3 bricks

4.5 ounces catfish, baked or grilled, with 1 tablespoon cocktail sauce

Creamy Coleslaw (page 216)

Water (no caffeine after 3:00 p.m.)

Snack—2 bricks

Recovery Shake (recipes start on page 223)

Day 6

Breakfast—3 bricks

3 ounces turkey sausage

¾ bran muffin with 2 teaspoons butter

1½ teaspoons cashew butter

Water, green tea, or coffee, with no sugar or milk

Snack—2 bricks

Recovery Shake (recipes start on page 223)

Lunch—3 bricks

Naked Taco Salad (page 201)

Water, green tea, or coffee, with no sugar or milk

Snack—2 bricks

3 ounces grilled chicken breast, 1 cup red bell pepper slices drizzled with 4½ teaspoons almond butter

Dinner—3 bricks

4.5 ounces cooked ground beef mixed with ⅓ cup tomato sauce, ½ cup green beans, and ¼ cup quinoa topped with 9 crushed almonds and 3 tablespoons sour cream

Water (no caffeine after 3:00 p.m.)

Snack—2 bricks

Recovery Shake (recipes start on page 223)

Day 7

Breakfast—3 bricks

6 egg whites, scrambled

½ cup cooked grits with 3 teaspoons butter

Water, green tea, or coffee, with no sugar or milk

Snack—2 bricks

Recovery Shake (recipes start on page 223)

Lunch—3 bricks

4.5 ounces canned tuna mixed with 9 tablespoons mashed avocado and served over ¾ cup kale and
  ⅓ cup chopped tomato drizzled with 1 tablespoon balsamic vinegar

Water, green tea, or coffee, with no sugar or milk

Snack—2 bricks

2 Badass Eggs (4 halves) (page 220)

Dinner—3 bricks

4.5 ounces salmon with 1 tablespoon cocktail sauce

18 steamed asparagus spears, drizzled with 1 tablespoon balsamic vinegar

3 teaspoons cream cheese on top of salmon

3 teaspoons almond butter

Water (no caffeine after 3:00 p.m.)

Snack—2 bricks

Recovery Shake (recipes start on page 223)

THE GAINER MENUS FOR FRAME 5 (CONFIDENT)

Remember that for each frame, you are permitted to eat within a range of bricks (see page 63). Adjust up and down within that range for your own needs. Feel free to substitute any meal with a Meal Replacement Shake (recipes start on page 227).

Week 1

Day 1

Breakfast—3 bricks
2 eggs, scrambled or poached, with 1 slice Canadian bacon
½ cup oatmeal cooked with 1 tablespoon raisins and 9 tablespoons half-and-half
Water, green tea, or coffee, with no sugar or milk

Snack—3 bricks
3 ounces canned tuna mixed with 1 tablespoon olive oil and served on 1 cup chopped tomato

Lunch—4 bricks
Chicken Vegetable Soup (page 197)
Water, green tea, or coffee, with no sugar or milk

Snack—2 bricks
Recovery Shake (recipes start on page 223)

Dinner—4 bricks
4 ounces sirloin steak
18 steamed asparagus spears, drizzled with 1 teaspoon melted butter
6 ounces mashed sweet potato, topped with 3 tablespoons sour cream and 7½ teaspoons bacon bits
Water (no caffeine after 3:00 p.m.)

Snack—2 bricks
Recovery Shake (recipes start on page 223)

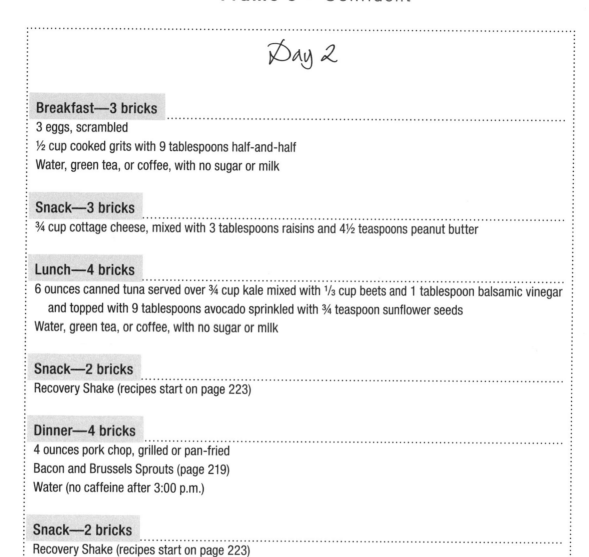

Day 2

Breakfast—3 bricks

3 eggs, scrambled

½ cup cooked grits with 9 tablespoons half-and-half

Water, green tea, or coffee, with no sugar or milk

Snack—3 bricks

¾ cup cottage cheese, mixed with 3 tablespoons raisins and 4½ teaspoons peanut butter

Lunch—4 bricks

6 ounces canned tuna served over ¾ cup kale mixed with ⅓ cup beets and 1 tablespoon balsamic vinegar and topped with 9 tablespoons avocado sprinkled with ¾ teaspoon sunflower seeds

Water, green tea, or coffee, with no sugar or milk

Snack—2 bricks

Recovery Shake (recipes start on page 223)

Dinner—4 bricks

4 ounces pork chop, grilled or pan-fried

Bacon and Brussels Sprouts (page 219)

Water (no caffeine after 3:00 p.m.)

Snack—2 bricks

Recovery Shake (recipes start on page 223)

Day 3

Breakfast—3 bricks

3 slices Canadian bacon, pan-fried

½ cup cooked grits with 1 teaspoon butter

3 teaspoons peanut butter

Water, green tea, or coffee, with no sugar or milk

Snack—3 bricks

3 hard-boiled eggs, ¾ apple, 4½ teaspoons peanut butter

Lunch—4 bricks

6 ounces cooked ground beef mixed with ⅓ cup tomato sauce, ¾ cup carrots, and ¼ cup cooked onion, topped with 3 tablespoons sour cream

4½ teaspoons almond butter

Water, green tea, or coffee, with no sugar or milk

Snack—2 bricks

Recovery Shake (recipes start on page 223)

Dinner—4 bricks

4 ounces veal chop

Zucchini Side Spaghetti (page 218)

8 macadamia nuts

Water (no caffeine after 3:00 p.m.)

Snack—2 bricks

Recovery Shake (recipes start on page 223)

Day 4

Breakfast—3 bricks

2 eggs scrambled with 1 ounce cubed ham

¾ cup oatmeal cooked with 4½ teaspoons peanut butter

Water, green tea, or coffee, with no sugar or milk

Snack—3 bricks

¾ cup cottage cheese, ¾ cup chopped fresh pineapple, 2¼ teaspoons sunflower seeds

Lunch—4 bricks

6 ounces ground turkey

½ cup cooked green beans, sprinkled with 18 crushed almonds and drizzled with 1 teaspoon melted
    butter

1 cup cooked carrots, drizzled with 1 teaspoon melted butter

6 tablespoons avocado

Water, green tea, or coffee, with no sugar or milk

Snack—2 bricks

Recovery Shake (recipes start on page 223)

Dinner—4 bricks

4 ounces grilled chicken breast

¾ cup cooked quinoa topped with ⅓ cup tomato sauce

½ avocado

Water (no caffeine after 3:00 p.m.)

Snack—2 bricks

Recovery Shake (recipes start on page 223)

Day 5

Breakfast—3 bricks

6 egg whites, scrambled

½ cup cooked oatmeal with 1 tablespoon raisins and 9 tablespoons half-and-half

Water, green tea, or coffee, with no sugar or milk

Snack—3 bricks

4.5 ounces canned tuna mixed with 3 tablespoon mayonnaise and served on 3 cups chopped tomato

Lunch—4 bricks

Spinach Salad (page 201)

Water, green tea, or coffee, with no sugar or milk

Snack—2 bricks

Recovery Shake (recipes start on page 223)

Dinner—4 bricks

6 ounces catfish, baked or grilled, with 1 tablespoon cocktail sauce

Creamy Coleslaw (page 216)

Water (no caffeine after 3:00 p.m.)

Snack—2 bricks

Recovery Shake (recipes start on page 223)

Day 6

Breakfast—3 bricks

3 ounces turkey sausage, pan-fried

¾ bran muffin with 2 teaspoons butter

1½ teaspoons peanut butter

Water, green tea, or coffee, with no sugar or milk

Snack—3 bricks

4.5 ounces grilled chicken breast, 1½ cups red bell pepper slices, 9 teaspoons cream cheese

Lunch—4 bricks

Naked Taco Salad (page 201)

Water, green tea, or coffee, with no sugar or milk

Snack—2 bricks

Recovery Shake (recipes start on page 223)

Dinner—4 bricks

6 ounces cooked ground beef mixed with ⅓ cup tomato sauce, ⅓ cup carrots, and 3 teaspoons cream cheese

½ cup butternut squash with 2 teaspoons butter

1½ teaspoons almond butter

Water (no caffeine after 3:00 p.m.)

Snack—2 bricks

Recovery Shake (recipes start on page 223)

Day 7

Breakfast—3 bricks

6 egg whites scrambled with ½ cup cooked mushrooms

9 ounces mashed sweet potato with 1 teaspoon butter topped with 3 teaspoons cream cheese

1½ teaspoons peanut butter

Water, green tea, or coffee, with no sugar or milk

Snack—3 bricks

3 Badass Eggs (6 halves) (page 220)

Lunch—4 bricks

6 ounces canned tuna mixed with 4 teaspoons olive oil and served over ¾ cup kale and ⅓ cup
   chopped tomato

½ cup blueberries

Water, green tea, or coffee, with no sugar or milk

Snack—2 bricks

Recovery Shake (recipes start on page 223)

Dinner—4 bricks

6 ounces salmon, pan-fried, with 1½ tablespoons tartar sauce

9 steamed asparagus spears, drizzled with 1 teaspoon butter

1 cup spaghetti squash topped with ⅓ cup tomato sauce and ¼ cup collard greens drizzled with
   6 teaspoons sour cream

Water (no caffeine after 3:00 p.m.)

Snack—2 bricks

Recovery Shake (recipes start on page 223)

I'M A BADASS

Alexia, age 31, competes in figure competitions and uses CrossFit to sculpt her body for them. Although she loves working out, she hit a wall with her training. She wasn't making any muscular gains, nor was she losing body fat.

"I knew Christmas had different diet plans for different body frames, so I wanted to see if these would work for me," Alexia said. "I had a competition four months away, so I had time to get in some major training if her diet worked."

Alexia started on the Maintainer plan. After 21 days, she moved into the Gainer category in order to add some weight on her lifts and build muscle mass. Three weeks prior to her competition, she used the Modifier plan to cut weight.

"Previously, I had always used drastic calorie-cutting approaches to leaning out for competition. They left me feeling malnourished and exhausted. This time it was different. With the Modifier plan, I easily burned off body fat, sculpted my body, and entered my competition feeling strong and confident."

The upshot of all this? Alexia took home a win with her new hot, curvy, strong look. Plus, she's lifting more weight than ever and setting new records in the gym.

"I now recommend this program to all my friends and training partners."

CHAPTER 10

The Badass Body Diet Recipes

I LOVE TO COOK, but like you, I'm busy, life happens. My workouts are grueling enough, so I sure don't like torturing myself with recipes that take too long and result in a sink loaded with dirty dishes. Preparing and cooking six meals a day can take up a lot of your precious time. At the same time, I want you to enjoy delicious food while following my Badass plan. So I've designed some amazing recipes that don't take a lot of time to make, which means minimal preparation but maximum flavor, from breakfasts to lunches to dinners, and snacks in between.

My recipes make from one to four servings. If you're living solo and not feeding a family, you can save the three extra servings as leftovers so you have meals prepared for several days. And most of my snacks, such as the Recovery Shakes, take seconds to whip up.

Some other timesaving tips for the time-crunched among us:

Plan ahead. Check my meal plans or the ones you devised for yourself. One day each week, make a grocery list based on your meal plan and head to the supermarket. Get all the foods you need for a week and stock your fridge and pantry. Trade plans with other Badass Bodies!

Have enough plastic bags and containers on hand. I use glass containers instead of plastic, but fall back on plastic bags when I need to. I use both of these to prepare and package my individual serving sizes for my bricks. I place my carb bricks on the top shelf of my fridge, the protein bricks on the middle shelf, and the rest of my food in the lower compartments. This level of organization may not be for you, but it can help make life less complicated and saves lots of time in the long run. Give it a TRY! You will be surprised at how easy this task makes this process.

Shop strategically. Purchase single-portion cuts of meat and fish, or ask the butcher to cut proteins into brick-sizes portions for you. Also, have the deli cut meat into slices to make measuring easy. If you buy prepackaged deli meat, determine how many slices make 7 grams of protein and divvy it up accordingly. I'll let you in on a secret: The 7-gram measurement usually turns out to be 1½ to 2 slices of turkey or ham.

Freeze any extras. Select fruits and vegetables by pieces instead of bagged produce that could go to waste. Frozen fruits and vegetables are handy; you can use them as needed.

Check out your local farmer's market. It offers the freshest, most seasonal food you can buy, and thus the highest in nutrients.

Regarding veggies: Buy frozen veggies and fruit over canned versions. Frozen veggies are often flash-frozen near the farm, meaning they were as ripe as possible before packaging. Their nutrient content is thus higher than canned foods or even veggies and fruit in the grocery store that are out of season and trucked long distances to get to your community. Veggies and fruit in the grocery store out of season (and sometimes in season) are often picked too early and have not yet ripened. That's a problem, since the produce may lack some major important nutrients.

Cook in bulk. Once you return home from the grocery store or the farmer's market, it's time to cook and measure your food. This is less daunting than you think. Here's how I do it:

Bulk-cook oven items together: chicken, sweet potatoes, veggies, and so forth. You can bake all the items together that run on the same temperature. Keep it simple.

Be a multitasker. While your chicken, sweet potatoes, and veggies are in the oven, cook up some other foods on the stovetop. For example, brown some ground turkey or hard-boil a batch of eggs. Also, start portioning out your fruit and sliced deli meat. Measure them into single bricks and separate them by bricks. Place them in containers and mark them, along with the number of bricks they contain. I do this for all my protein and carb foods that I'll be eating for the week, with the exception of meals I plan to cook fresh for dinner. The result is that the fridge is full of individual serving sizes of bricks to help me pick and choose the foods I want that day without having the hassle of measuring it when I'm on a tight schedule.

Once the food in the oven and on the stovetop is done, you can measure it out and put it into individually marked brick containers too, or freeze food for meals later in the week. At mealtimes, just reheat desired portion or portions and enjoy—while you lose weight.

From making out my grocery list to shopping to food prepping and cooking, this entire process takes me less than two hours.

Carry a ready-to-drink Recovery Shake with you to the gym. That way, you get your shake in within that 10-minute window of working out. This makes it easier for the body to get nutrients for muscle building and fat burning. Meal Replacement Shakes also help you avoid feeling hungry throughout the day and therefore overeating.

Spice it up. Cut back on salt and experiment with different herbs, spices, and seasonings to enhance flavor. Some of my favorites: sautéing garlic in a very small amount of oil or squeezing lemon juice over fish or veggies. Find other ways to add flavor, such as marinating meats in tomato juice or chicken broth before you cook them.

Employ healthy cooking techniques. Try methods like oven frying over deep frying using gallons of oil. You can oven-fry fish, poultry, shellfish, and meatballs by coating them with a pulverized nut coating, spritzing them with vegetable oil cooking spray, and then baking. The dish will come out tasty and crispy. I love to use nonstick cookware too. It makes it easier to use less oil and keeps food from sticking (which helps cut down on cleanup time). I also love to steam my food, especially veggies, because it seals moisture in food. I use a steaming basket over the stovetop or a specialty steamer appliance. Grilling is another of my favorite ways to cook; it doesn't require a lot of added fat and adds a nice smoky flavor.

I encourage you to try as many of these recipes as you can—even if you think you hate cooking or don't know how to cook (if you can read and follow instructions, you can cook!).

See you in the kitchen!

Hip Advice: Get Creative in the Kitchen with Combo Meals

In addition to following recipes, try to create your own. It's really easy with what I call combo cooking. A combo dish is anything that has a protein, carbohydrate, and often, a fat in it. Some examples are chili, soups, and casseroles. Be sure to add fat to your meal to customize it for your meal plan.

One of my favorite combo meals is chili. I like to start by cooking 10 bricks of ground turkey and adding 10 bricks of a mix of carbohydrates.

I measure out 10 bricks of these carbs (including the tomato paste) with all my favorite dry seasoning and throw it into the pot with the cooked ground turkey. For primo carbs, I use a tomato paste (with some added water), broccoli, zucchini, squash, onions, and any other in-season veggie I can get my hands on (I don't use beans or peas). The veggies cook down, and you end up with a hearty chili with tons of flavor!

I pull out my containers—usually five—to prepare 2-brick servings of my chili. I store it for my lunches or dinners later or enjoy a serving that night. I prefer to add the fat when I eat it. For a fat, I love black olives mixed into the chili. Another favorite is sour cream.

Approach any of these combo items the same way. It's best to have a 1:1 ratio of protein and carbs for simplicity then you will need to add the fat to the meal before eating. Adjust any recipe to balance out the carbohydrates or proteins as needed. Not all recipes will be exactly balanced bricks.

MEXICAN OMELET

1 serving

Olive oil cooking spray
½ cup chopped green pepper
¼ jalapeño pepper, seeded and diced
¼ cup chopped onion
2 eggs
1 teaspoon olive oil
Salt and pepper to taste

Spray a small skillet with olive oil cooking spray. Sauté the peppers and onion over medium heat until just tender. Remove the vegetables to a small plate.

In a bowl, whisk the eggs and olive oil with 2 tablespoons of water and olive oil. Season with salt and pepper.

Respray the skillet you used to sauté the vegetables. Pour the egg mixture into the skillet and heat over medium heat. Cook the eggs, using a spatula to allow uncooked egg to run underneath cooked egg. When the omelet is set, spoon the vegetable mixture over half of it. Fold the omelet in half over the vegetable mixture. Cover and cook for 1 minute.

Nutrition: 2 bricks. To create a 3-brick omelet, increase to ¾ cup green pepper, ½ jalapeño, ½ cup onion, 3 eggs, and ½ teaspoon olive oil.

MINI QUICHE

1 serving

Olive oil cooking spray
½ cup chopped onion
2 cups chopped fresh spinach
2 eggs
2 teaspoons olive oil
Salt and pepper, to taste

Preheat the oven to 350 degrees F.

Spray a small skillet with olive oil cooking spray. Sauté the onion and spinach over medium heat until just tender. Remove the vegetables to a small plate.

Whisk the eggs in a bowl with the olive oil. Season with salt and pepper to taste. Add the vegetable mixture and mix well.

Spray a small ramekin with cooking spray. Pour the egg and vegetable mixture into the ramekin. Bake for 20 minutes, or until the quiche is set.

Nutrition: 2 bricks. To create a 3-brick quiche, increase to ¾ cup onion, 3 cups spinach, 3 eggs, and 1 teaspoon olive oil.

GRAIN-FREE GRANOLA

1 serving

6 crushed almonds
2 tablespoons unsweetened shredded coconut
1 teaspoon chia seeds
1 tablespoon dried cranberries
¼ teaspoon ground cinnamon
Coconut water or almond milk

Mix all the ingredients except the coconut water or almond milk to a cereal bowl and mix well. Moisten with coconut water or almond milk to taste.

Nutrition: 2 bricks. To create a 3-brick cereal, increase recipe to 9 crushed almonds, 2 tablespoons cranberries, and 3 tablespoons shredded coconut.

CHICKEN VEGETABLE SOUP

2 servings

¼ cup chopped onion
2 celery stalks, chopped
1 carrot, chopped
¼ head of cabbage, shredded
½ cup canned tomato puree
2 cups chicken or vegetable stock, plus more as needed
2 teaspoons olive oil
½ teaspoon garlic powder
Salt and pepper to taste
1 cup diced baked chicken breast

Place all the ingredients except the chopped chicken in a medium saucepan over medium heat. Bring to a boil, then reduce the heat, cover, and simmer until the vegetables are tender, about 15 to 20 minutes. Add more broth if needed as you cook. Add the chicken and heat it through. Adjust seasonings if necessary.

Nutrition: 3 bricks per serving. To create a 4-brick soup, increase to ½ cup onion, 2 carrots, ¾ cup tomato puree, 1 tablespoon olive oil, and 1¼ cups chopped chicken.

TEXAS-STYLE CHILI

2 servings

3 ounces ground beef
2 ounces ground turkey sausage
½ onion, chopped
1 garlic clove, minced
1 cup chopped green pepper
1 cup canned diced stewed tomatoes (do not drain)
1 tablespoon chili powder
1 teaspoon ground cumin
Salt and pepper to taste

In a medium skillet, brown the beef and turkey sausage over medium-high heat until well-done, with no pink in the meat. Place the meat mixture in a medium saucepan and add the remaining ingredients. Simmer over low heat until the vegetables are tender and the chili has thickened slightly, about 15 to 20 minutes.

Nutrition: 3 bricks per serving. To create a 4-brick soup, increase to 5 ounces ground beef, 5 ounces ground turkey sausage, and 1 onion.

STUFFED TOMATO WITH CRAB SALAD

1 serving

1 cup canned crabmeat (about two 4-ounce cans), drained
1 celery stalk, minced
2 black olives, minced
1 tablespoon olive oil
⅛ teaspoon Old Bay seasoning
Salt to taste
2 cups shredded lettuce
1 large tomato, quartered

In a medium bowl, combine the crabmeat, celery, olives, oil, Old Bay, and salt. Lay the lettuce on a plate and top with the tomatoes and crab mixture.

Nutrition: 3 bricks per serving. To create a 4-brick salad, increase to 1⅓ cups crabmeat, 3 black olives, 1 teaspoon olive oil, and 2 tomatoes.

SWEET TUNA SALAD

1 serving

One 3-ounce can water-packed tuna, drained
½ apple, peeled and chopped
1 tablespoon olive oil
Salt to taste
2 cups shredded lettuce

In a medium bowl, combine the tuna, apple, olive oil, and salt to taste. Arrange the lettuce on a plate and top with the tuna salad.

Nutrition: 3 bricks per serving (1). To create a 4-brick salad, increase to 4 ounces tuna, 1 apple, and 1 extra teaspoon olive oil.

CHICKEN WRAPS

1 serving

2.5 ounces skinless boneless chicken breast, baked or grilled ahead of time, then chopped into ½-inch cubes
15 grapes, halved
2 celery stalks, chopped
1 tablespoon olive oil
Salt and pepper to taste
2 or 3 large lettuce leaves

In a medium bowl, combine the chopped chicken, grapes, celery, olive oil, and salt and pepper. Scoop some chicken mixture onto each lettuce leaf. Roll up and enjoy.

Nutrition: 3 bricks. To create 4-brick wraps, increase to 3.5 ounces chicken, 22 grapes, and 1 extra teaspoon olive oil.

NAKED TACO SALAD

1 serving

2.5 ounces cooked ground turkey (pan-fry until cooked throughout)
¼ cup chopped green or jalapeño pepper
½ cup salsa
2 cups shredded lettuce
2 tablespoons sour cream

In a small bowl, combine the cooked turkey, pepper, and salsa. Serve over the lettuce and top with the sour cream.

Nutrition: 3 bricks. To create a 4-brick salad, increase to 3.5 ounces turkey, 1 cup salsa, and 1 extra teaspoon sour cream (for a total of 2 tablespoons + 1 teaspoon).

SPINACH SALAD

4 servings

6 to 8 ounces feta cheese
8 cups baby spinach leaves
2 cups chopped tomato
2 cucumbers, chopped
3 tablespoons raisins
½ cup plus 2 tablespoons bacon bits or chopped cooked bacon
Balsamic Dressing (see page 216)

In a large bowl, gently toss the feta, spinach, tomato, cucumbers, raisins, and bacon bits until well combined. Arrange the salad on plates and drizzle with Balsamic Dressing (about 1 tablespoon per salad).

Nutrition: 3 bricks per serving. To create a 4-brick recipe, increase to 18 ounces of cheese, 5 tablespoons raisins, and 2 tablespoons dressing.

BLACKENED WHITEFISH

4 servings

2 tablespoons smoked paprika
2 teaspoons onion powder
½ teaspoon cayenne pepper
1 teaspoon freshly ground black pepper
½ teaspoon kosher salt
1½ pounds fresh fish fillets, such as tilapia, cod, or perch
Olive oil cooking spray

Combine all the spices in a small bowl and mix well.

Rub the spice mixture into the fish fillets. Let sit for 30 minutes (no longer) at room temperature for the flavors to soak in.

Coat a large skillet with olive oil cooking spray. Place the fillets in the skillet and pan-fry over medium-high heat for about 3 minutes on each side, or until the fish flakes easily with a fork and is cooked through.

Nutrition: A 3-ounce cooked serving of this dish will provide the right amount of protein for a 3-brick dinner (along with the carbohydrate and fat you choose to complement the fish); a 4-ounce cooked serving will provide the right amount of protein for a 4-brick dinner.

"SMOKED" SALMON

4 servings

Vegetable oil cooking spray
1½ pounds fresh salmon fillets
1 tablespoon Liquid Smoke
Kosher salt, to taste
½ to ¾ cup chopped fresh dill

Preheat the oven to 400 degrees F.

Spray a glass baking dish with vegetable oil cooking spray and arrange the fillets in the dish. Brush Liquid Smoke generously over the salmon and sprinkle it with salt. Cover the fish liberally with dill and bake for 20 to 30 minutes, or until the salmon flakes easily with a fork.

Nutrition: A 3.5-ounce cooked serving of this dish will provide the right amount of protein for a 3-brick dinner (along with the carbohydrate and fat you choose to complement the fish); a 4.5-ounce cooked serving will provide the right amount of protein for a 4-brick dinner.

SHRIMP SCAMPI

4 servings

1 tablespoon olive oil
1½ pounds large shrimp, peeled and deveined
4 garlic cloves, minced
2 tablespoons fresh-squeezed lemon juice
½ teaspoon dried Italian seasoning
Salt and pepper to taste

Heat the oil in a large skillet over medium heat. Add the shrimp and sauté until opaque, 2 to 4 minutes. Add the rest of the ingredients and cook for another 1 or 2 minutes, or until the garlic is softened.

Nutrition: 3 bricks. A 3.5-ounce cooked serving of this dish will provide the right amount of protein for a 3-brick dinner (along with the carbohydrate you choose to complement the fish); a 4.5-ounce cooked serving will provide the right amount of protein for a 4-brick dinner. Add 1 extra teaspoon of olive oil for a 4-brick dinner.

COCONUT SHRIMP

4 servings

Olive oil cooking spray
¼ cup almond flour (or ½ cup almonds ground in the blender)
1 teaspoon salt
¼ cup unsweetened shredded coconut
1 pound large shrimp, peeled and deveined
3 egg whites, beaten
1 pound large shrimp, peeled and deveined

Preheat the oven to 400 degrees F and lightly coat a baking sheet with olive oil cooking spray.

Combine the almond flour and salt in a shallow bowl. Place the coconut in a separate shallow bowl. In a third bowl, lightly beat or whisk the egg whites. Dredge one shrimp at a time in the almond flour, then in the egg whites. Finally, roll the shrimp in the coconut, coating well. Place on the baking sheet. Repeat with the rest of the shrimp.

Spray the shrimp liberally with cooking spray. Bake for 12 to 15 minutes, or until the coconut is lightly browned, turning the shrimp halfway through.

Nutrition: A 3-ounce serving of this dish will provide the right amount of protein for a 3-brick dinner (along with the carbohydrate and fat you choose to complement the fish); a 4-ounce serving will provide the right amount of protein for a 4-brick dinner. Each serving provides approximately 1 gram of carbohydrate and 6 grams of fat (the amount of fat found in 4 bricks).

BACON-WRAPPED SEA SCALLOPS

4 servings

20 large (jumbo) sea scallops (5 scallops per serving; each scallop weighs about ½ ounce)
10 slices uncooked bacon
Olive oil cooking spray
Garlic powder to taste
Salt to taste
Lemon pepper to taste

Preheat the oven to 425 degrees F.

Wrap each scallop in ½ strip of bacon and secure it with a toothpick. Spray lightly with olive oil cooking spray and sprinkle with the seasonings.

Place the scallops in a glass baking dish and bake 8 minutes on one side, then 8 minutes on the other side. Make sure that the bacon is nearly crisp and the scallops are cooked through and opaque. Drain the scallops on a paper towel prior to serving.

Nutrition: A 5-scallop serving of this dish will provide the right amount of protein and fat for a 3-brick dinner (along with the carbohydrate you choose to complement the fish); a 6-scallop serving will provide approximately the right amount of protein and fat for a 4-brick dinner.

NUDE CHICKEN FAJITAS

4 servings

1½ tablespoons olive oil
10 ounces boneless skinless chicken breasts, cut into thin strips
1 green bell pepper, cut into ½-inch slices
1 red bell pepper, cut into ½-inch slices
1 yellow bell pepper, cut into ½-inch slices
1 white onion, cut into ½-inch slices
4 garlic cloves, minced
1 tablespoon chili powder
1 teaspoon ground cumin
Salt and pepper to taste
Lettuce leaves
½ cup salsa

In a large skillet over medium-high heat, heat the olive oil. Add the chicken strips and sauté until cooked through, about 10 to 15 minutes. Don't overcook the chicken or it will be rubbery. Add the vegetables and spices and sauté until the vegetables are tender, another 2 minutes.

Arrange lettuce leaves on four plates. Top with the fajita mixture and serve with salsa.

Nutrition: 3 bricks per serving. To create a 4-brick recipe, increase to 2 tablespoons olive oil, 12 ounces chicken, 2 green bell peppers, 2 red bell peppers, and 1 cup salsa.

TURKEY LOAF

4 servings

Olive oil cooking spray
1 pound ground turkey
⅓ cup almonds, processed to a fine flour in a blender or food processor
2 eggs, well beaten
1 onion, diced
2 carrots, shredded
1 red bell pepper, chopped
4 garlic cloves, minced
⅓ cup tomato paste
2 teaspoons salt
½ teaspoon pepper

Preheat the oven to 400 degrees F and coat a loaf pan with olive oil cooking spray.

In a large bowl, combine all the ingredients well. Form the mixture into a loaf in the prepared pan. Bake for about 1 hour, or until cooked through.

Nutrition: 3 bricks per serving. To create a 4-brick recipe, increase to 20 ounces turkey, ½ cup almonds, 3 eggs, 2 red bell peppers, and ⅔ cup tomato paste.

"SPAGHETTI" AND MEATBALLS

4 servings

"Spaghetti"
Olive oil cooking spray
1 large spaghetti squash (four ¾-cup servings)

Meatballs
1 pound ground turkey
½ cup finely chopped onion
4 garlic cloves, minced
¼ cup minced fresh basil leaves
½ zucchini, shredded
2 eggs, well beaten
⅓ cup almonds, processed to a fine flour in a blender or food processor
2 teaspoons salt
½ teaspoon pepper
1 cup no-sugar-added marinara sauce, such as Monte Bene Spicy Marinara

Preheat the oven to 400 degrees F and coat a baking sheet with olive oil cooking spray.

Cut the squash in half and remove seeds. Place the halves cut side down in a glass baking dish. Fill the dish with water up to ½ inch. Bake for 45 minutes, or until the squash is tender. Remove the spaghetti-like strands from the squash and keep them warm.

Meanwhile, combine all the ingredients for the meatballs in a large bowl and mix well with your hands. Form the mixture into Ping-Pong-size balls and place them an inch or so apart on the prepared baking sheet. Bake for about 30 minutes, until browned and cooked through.

Serve the meatballs over the squash "spaghetti" and top with marinara sauce.

Nutrition: 3 bricks per serving. To create a 4-brick recipe, increase recipe to 18 ounces turkey, 4 cups marinara sauce, 3 eggs, and ½ cup almonds.

STUFFED PEPPERS

4 servings

Olive oil cooking spray
4 large red or green bell peppers
1 pound lean ground beef
½ cup chopped onion
2 teaspoons garlic powder
1 egg, beaten
¼ cup almonds, processed to a fine flour in a blender or food processor
2 teaspoons dried Italian seasoning
Salt and pepper to taste
1 cup no-sugar-added marinara sauce, such as Monte Bene Spicy Marinara

Preheat the oven to 350 degrees F and spray a glass baking dish with olive oil cooking spray.

Cut the tops off the bell peppers. Place the peppers in a pot of salted boiling water for about 5 minutes, or until slightly softened. Drain them well.

In a large skillet, brown the ground beef. Drain. Combine the beef with the remaining ingredients (except the marinara sauce). Fill the peppers with the meat mixture. Place the peppers in the prepared baking dish and spoon sauce over each pepper.

Cover the dish with foil. Bake the peppers for 30 to 45 minutes.

Nutrition: 3 bricks per serving. To create a 4-brick recipe, increase recipe to 20 ounces ground beef, ⅓ cup almonds, and 2 cups marinara sauce.

CROCKED POT ROAST

4 servings

1½- to 2-pound chuck roast
6 garlic cloves
1 onion, chopped
½ cup sweet red wine, rosé, or Moscato
One 14.5-ounce can diced tomatoes
Salt and pepper to taste

Using a knife, make 6 slits at various places in the roast. Insert the garlic cloves into the slits.

Place the onion, wine, and tomatoes in a slow cooker. Add the roast and salt and pepper it generously. Cover and cook on high for 4 to 5 hours, or until the roast is very tender.

Nutrition: 3 bricks per serving; each serving of meat should weigh 3 ounces. To create a 4-brick recipe, use 4-ounce servings of meat.

LOW-CARB LOVERS' PIZZA

4 servings

"Crust"
Olive oil cooking spray
1 pound ground beef
½ cup chopped onion
1 teaspoon garlic powder
1 egg, beaten

Toppings
1 cup sliced mushrooms
1 cup chopped green or red bell pepper
½ cup chopped onion
1½ cups no-sugar-added marinara sauce, such as Monte Bene Spicy Marinara
1 teaspoon dried Italian seasoning
Salt and pepper to taste

Preheat the oven to 450 degrees F and spray a 16-inch pizza pan with olive oil cooking spray.

In a large bowl, combine the beef, onion, garlic powder, and egg. Spread the mixture out on the prepared pan. Bake for 10 to 15 minutes, or until the meat is brown throughout and well-done. Drain off the juices.

While the "crust" is baking, spray a large skillet with olive oil cooking spray. Add the mushrooms, bell pepper, and onion and sauté until tender, about 5 minutes.

Preheat the broiler.

Spread the marinara sauce over the crust. Top with the sautéed vegetables and seasonings. Broil the pizza until the top turns slightly brown, about 5 minutes (watch it carefully).

Cut the pizza into 4 slices and serve.

Nutrition: 3 bricks per serving. To create a 4-brick recipe, cut the pizza into thirds rather than fourths.

SMOTHERED PORK CHOPS

4 servings

Olive oil cooking spray
4 small boneless pork chops (2½ to 3 ounces each)
Salt and pepper to taste
3 apples, cored and sliced
1 tablespoon vegetable oil
½ teaspoon apple pie spice

Spray a large skillet with olive oil cooking spray. Add the pork chops and season with salt and pepper. Pan-fry over medium heat for about 5 minutes on each side, or until cooked through. Set the pork chops aside.

Place the apples and oil in a smaller skillet and sprinkle with apple pie spice. Sauté the apples until soft, about 5 to 6 minutes.

Serve the pork chops topped with the apples.

Nutrition: 3 bricks per serving. To create a 4-brick recipe, use 4-ounce pork chops, 2 tablespoons vegetable oil, and 4 apples.

HERB-ROASTED LAMB

4 servings

12 ounces lamb, such as a loin roast cut or tenderloin
4 garlic cloves, halved
1 tablespoon plus 1 teaspoon olive oil
1 teaspoon garlic powder
1 tablespoon chopped fresh rosemary
1 teaspoon dried thyme
1 teaspoon salt
¼ teaspoon pepper

Preheat the oven to 325 degrees F.

With a small knife, make 8 tiny incisions evenly over the meat; insert the garlic halves. Rub the lamb with the oil.

In a small bowl, combine the garlic powder, rosemary, thyme, salt, and pepper. Rub the mixture over the lamb.

Place the lamb in a roasting pan and roast it for up to 1 hour, or until meat thermometer inserted in the thickest part of the lamb registers 145°F to 165°F, depending on how well done you want it.

Nutrition: 3 bricks per serving. To create a 4-brick recipe, use about 14 ounces lamb and 2 tablespoons vegetable oil. Complement the dish with your choice of a primo carb.

ITALIAN SALAD

4 servings

4 medium tomatoes (such as Roma), quartered
½ white onion, quartered and thinly sliced
½ cup chopped fresh basil leaves
Salt and pepper to taste
Balsamic Dressing (recipe below)

In a large bowl, toss the tomatoes, onion, basil, and salt and pepper to taste. Serve on four salad plates and drizzle each with 1 to 1½ tablespoons Balsamic Dressing.

Nutrition: One serving provides 7 grams of primo carbs. One tablespoon of dressing provides 4.5 grams of fat; 1½ tablespoons provides 6 grams of fat.

BALSAMIC DRESSING

Makes 1½ cups

½ cup white balsamic vinegar
½ teaspoon garlic powder
½ teaspoon onion powder
1 teaspoon dried Italian seasoning

1 teaspoon salt
½ teaspoon pepper
Pinch of cayenne pepper
1 cup olive oil

Place the vinegar and 2 tablespoons water in a jar with a lid. Add the seasonings. Place the lid on the jar and shake well. Add the oil and shake well until you have a smooth dressing. You can store this in your refrigerator for up to 3 weeks.

CREAMY COLESLAW

4 servings

4 cups shredded raw cabbage
¼ cup olive oil

¼ cup fresh-squeezed lemon juice
Salt and pepper to taste

In a large bowl, toss all the ingredients until well combined. Chill before serving.

Nutrition: One serving provides 9 grams of primo carbs and 5 grams of fat.

SAUTÉED GREENS

4 servings

1 tablespoon olive oil
Two 5-ounce bags baby spinach
One 5-ounce bag baby kale
4 garlic cloves, minced
2 tablespoons chopped fresh rosemary
Salt and pepper to taste

Heat the oil in a large skillet over medium heat. Add the greens, herbs, and salt and pepper and sauté until tender, about 8 to 10 minutes.

Nutrition: One serving provides 8 grams of primo carbs and 4 grams of fat.

ZUCCHINI SIDE SPAGHETTI

4 servings

4 zucchini
2 yellow summer squash
2 teaspoons salt, plus more to taste
1 garlic clove, minced
2 tablespoons olive oil
Pepper, to taste
1 cup no-sugar-added marinara sauce, such as Monte Bene Spicy Marinara

Cut the zucchini and squash into thin, noodle-like strips. You can use a knife, or better yet, a handy little tool called a spiralizer (available at kitchen stores or online). Toss the "noodles" with salt and place them in a colander to drain for at least 30 minutes.

Bring a pot of water to boil. Add the zucchini and squash "noodles" and cook for 1 minute. Drain, then rinse with cold water.

Heat the oil in a large skillet over medium-high heat. Add the zucchini, squash, and garlic and sauté until just tender, about 5 minutes. Season as desired with salt and pepper. Serve the "noodles" topped with warm marinara sauce.

Nutrition: One serving provides 16 grams of primo carbs and 6.5 grams of fat.

BACON AND BRUSSELS SPROUTS

4 servings

1 cup chicken broth
3 garlic cloves, minced
1½ pounds fresh Brussels sprouts, halved
5 slices bacon

Combine the broth, garlic, and Brussels sprouts in a medium saucepan. Cover and cook over medium heat until the Brussels sprouts are tender, 12 to 14 minutes. Drain the liquid from the pan.

While the Brussels sprouts are cooking, place the bacon in a large skillet and cook over medium-high heat until slightly crisp. Drain the bacon on paper towels and break it into ¼-inch pieces.

Mix the bacon into the Brussels sprouts and serve.

Nutrition: One serving provides 16 grams of primo carbs and 4.5 grams of fat.

BADASS EGGS

8 deviled egg halves

4 hard-boiled eggs
6 tablespoons mashed avocado
1 teaspoon olive oil
Salt and pepper to taste

Cut the eggs in half and carefully remove the yolks to a medium bowl. To the yolks, add the avocado, oil, and salt and pepper to taste and mix until well combined. Fill each halved egg white with the yolk and avocado mixture.

Nutrition: One serving (2 halves) provides 7 grams of primo protein and 4.5 grams of fat. Add 10 grams of carb and you have a perfect 1-brick snack.

Hip Advice: How to Make Perfect Hard-Boiled Eggs

Place eggs in a saucepan and cover with water. Place the pan over high heat and bring to a boil. When the water begins to boil, lower heat to medium and let eggs simmer for exactly 12 minutes. Drain off the hot water and run cold water over the eggs or cover with ice water until eggs are cool to the touch. Peel or refrigerate. Either way, you'll have hard-boiled eggs that peel perfectly.

EGG MUFFIN SNACKS

4 snacks

Olive oil cooking spray
4 eggs
⅓ cup cooked bacon (about 3 slices) (cook bacon until crispy, then crumble it)
¼ cup diced jalapeño pepper
1 tablespoon olive oil
Salt and pepper to taste

Preheat the oven to 350 degrees F and coat 4 cups of a muffin tin with olive oil cooking spray.

In a medium bowl, lightly whisk the eggs. Add the crumbled bacon, jalapeño pepper, olive oil, and salt and pepper and mix well. Divide the mixture evenly among the 4 muffin tins.

Bake for 18 to 20 minutes, or until a knife inserted into one of the muffins comes out clean. Cool, then refrigerate for snacks later.

Nutrition: One serving provides 7 grams of primo protein and 4.5 grams of fat. Add 10 grams of carb and you have a perfect 1-brick snack.

ZUCCHINI CHIPS

About 2 cups

Olive oil cooking spray
2 large zucchini, cut into ¼-inch rounds
2 tablespoons olive oil
Garlic powder to taste
Kosher salt to taste

Preheat the oven to 225 degrees F and coat 2 large baking sheets with olive oil cooking spray.

Spread the zucchini rounds in a single layer on paper towels. Cover the rounds with more paper towels and gently press down to extract as much liquid as possible.

Place the zucchini rounds in a single layer on the prepared baking sheets. Brush them with olive oil and sprinkle lightly with garlic powder and kosher salt.

Bake until the zucchini chips are browned and crisp, about 2 hours. Cool before serving. Store in an airtight container for up to 3 days.

Nutrition: Each ½-cup serving provides 6 grams of primo carbs and 7 grams of fat.

RECOVERY SHAKE AND MEAL REPLACEMENT SHAKES . . . KNOW THE DIFFERENCE.

There is a major difference between Recovery Shakes and Meal Replacement Shakes. Recovery shakes are generally only for post workout and should be consumed within 10 minutes of completing your workout, before you cool down. These do not have any fat in them so your body can utilize the nutrients in them immediately.

Meal Replacement Shakes are meals with a balanced amount of the macronutrients—protein, carbohydrate, and fat. These can be consumed to replace any meal—breakfast, lunch, or dinner—or snack. Understand your body category and which ones apply to you.

Below are a few of my favorite recipes!

RECOVERY SHAKES

Here are several Recovery Shakes you can use in the plan where suggested. Feel free to use the ones you like best, but try them all for variety.

BASIC BOOTY RECOVERY SHAKE

1 serving

½ scoop vanilla whey protein powder
1 cup almond milk
⅓ cup fresh or frozen berries

Place all the ingredients in a blender and blend until smooth.

Nutrition: This is a 1-brick recovery shake. For a 2-brick shake, increase to 1 scoop whey protein, ⅔ cup fresh or frozen berries.

TROPICAL GREEN SMOOTHIE

1 serving

½ scoop vanilla whey protein powder
1 cup almond milk
¼ frozen banana
1 handful fresh spinach

Place all the ingredients in a blender and blend until smooth.

Nutrition: This is a 1-brick recovery shake. For a 2-brick shake, increase to 1 scoop whey protein, 1½ cups almond milk, ½ frozen banana.

CHOCOLATE SMOOTHIE

1 serving

½ scoop chocolate whey protein powder
1 cup almond milk
⅓ cup coconut water

Place all the ingredients in a blender and blend until smooth.

Nutrition: This is a 1-brick recovery shake. For a 2-brick shake, increase to 1 scoop whey protein, 1½ cups almond milk, ⅔ cup coconut water.

CANDY BAR SMOOTHIE

1 serving

½ scoop vanilla whey protein powder
1 tablespoon unsweetened cocoa powder or cacao powder
1 cup almond milk
⅓ cup coconut water
¼ teaspoon pure vanilla extract

Place all the ingredients in a blender and blend until smooth.

Nutrition: This is a 1-brick recovery shake. For a 2-brick shake, increase to 1 scoop whey protein, 1½ tablespoons cocoa or cacao powder, 1½ cups almond milk, ½ cup coconut water.

STRAWBERRY SHORTCAKE SMOOTHIE

1 serving

½ scoop vanilla whey protein powder

1 cup almond milk

⅓ cup fresh or frozen chopped strawberries

¼ teaspoon pure vanilla extract

Place all the ingredients in a blender and blend until smooth.

Nutrition: This is a 1-brick recovery shake. For a 2-brick shake, increase to 1 scoop whey protein, 1½ cups almond milk, ⅔ cup berries.

PIÑA COLADA SMOOTHIE

1 serving

¼ cup fresh or frozen pineapple chunks

¼ frozen chopped banana

1 scoop vanilla whey protein powder

1 cup almond milk

2 teaspoons unsweetened coconut flakes as garnish, optional

Place the pineapple, banana, vanilla whey protein, and almond milk in a blender and blend until smooth. Garnish with coconut flakes, if desired.

Nutrition: This is a 2-brick recovery shake.

MEAL REPLACEMENT SHAKES

With your Meal Replacement Shake it's fine—and indeed a good idea—to toss a handful of fresh spinach or kale into any one of these meal replacers. You may use these to replace any breakfast, lunch, or dinner—for convenience and a quick meal when you're crunched for time—on any of the four Badass plans. Be sure to adjust the quantities of ingredients and fat amount to accommodate your need for your brick. All shakes below are measured as a Maintainer or Gainer.

SUPER STRAWBERRY SHAKE

1 serving

1 scoop strawberry whey protein powder
1 cup almond milk

2 cups frozen chopped strawberries
6 tablespoons half-and-half

Place all the ingredients in a blender and blend until smooth.

CHOCOLATE BANANA DREAM

1 serving

1 scoop chocolate whey protein powder
1 cup almond milk

½ frozen banana, cut into small pieces
3 teaspoons almond butter

Place all the ingredients in a blender and blend until smooth.

BLACK FOREST SMOOTHIE

2 servings

1 scoop chocolate whey protein powder
1 cup whole milk
½ cup frozen cherries
3 teaspoons peanut butter

Place all the ingredients in a blender and blend until smooth.

ISLAND TIME SHAKE

1 serving

1 scoop vanilla whey protein powder
1 cup almond milk
¾ cup frozen mango pieces
2 tablespoons shredded or flaked coconut, unsweetened
3 teaspoons almond butter

Place all the ingredients in a blender and blend until smooth.

CHERRY BERRY SMOOTHIE

3 servings

1½ scoops vanilla or strawberry protein powder
1 cup whole milk
½ cup frozen chopped strawberries
½ cup frozen cherries
2 tablespoons shredded or flaked coconut, unsweetened
9 tablespoons half-and-half

Place all the ingredients in a blender and blend until smooth.

BLUEBERRY DELIGHT

2 servings

½ scoop vanilla whey protein powder
1 cup whole milk
½ cup frozen blueberries
3 teaspoons almond butter

Place all the ingredients in a blender and blend until smooth.

PART 3

THE 12 MINUTES OF CHRISTMAS: WORK YOUR BUTT OFF

CHAPTER 11

Better Your Booty with Ass-tounding Exercises

BEAUTIFYING YOUR BOOTY—THAT'S OUR top goal here. I've shown you how to do it with diet. Now it's time to improve the shape and tone of your glutes with killer moves that will fire up your muscle fibers and stimulate positive changes.

Thanks to genetics, the butt is where most of us store fat, which can make it harder to tone. And very few of us have ready access to an airbrush to tidy up those less-than-perfect photos. But luckily, I know how to clear away any obstacle, genetic or otherwise, to getting your glutes in gear. With the moves you'll learn here, you'll see serious results. You'll get faster results too, because these exercises involve multiple muscle groups and force your heart to work harder—and that translates into a great fat burn.

I'm thrilled to share the booty and body exercises that helped me become a fitness athlete and model—and the ones that convinced me to toss out my baggy sweatpants and wear those hot Brazilian suits when I'm at the beach or by the pool.

Be consistent with these exercises, and work on perfecting your form. Safety is paramount. As a general rule, don't hold your breath during this exercise. Holding your breath will interfere with your physical energy. Always breathe naturally while exercising. Keep your tummy tight and "engaged" during the entire workout no matter what. Then follow the routines in the next chapter, and you'll be pleased with what you see in the mirror.

JUMPING JACKS

The Payoff: This exercise burns calories to help with weight loss and management, improves your cardiovascular endurance, and strengthens and tones your muscles all over. Perform jumping jacks before a vigorous activity or workout to warm up your muscles.

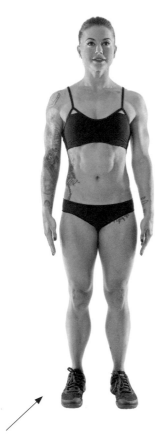

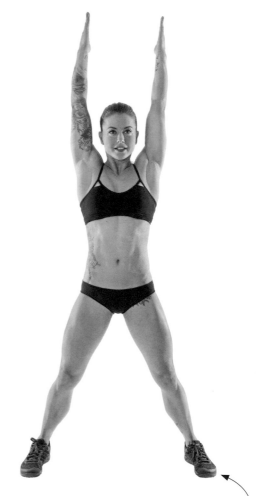

Begin in standing position, with your feet about a foot apart and your arms at your sides.

Simultaneously raise your arms overhead and spread your legs out to the sides. Land on the balls of your feet with your legs apart and with a slight bend in your knees to absorb the shock.

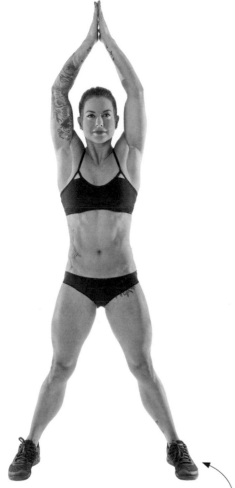

Where It Burns: In your thighs, tummy, and calves.

Blunders to Avoid: Do not bend your elbows; keep your arms straight throughout the move.

Tip: Use jumping jacks as a cool way to squeeze some heart-pumping cardio into your day without having to go to the gym or spend hours exercising. Jumping jacks can be performed during breaks, while watching TV, virtually anywhere.

Clap your hands over your head. Immediately jump again and return your arms and legs to the starting position to finish one full jumping jack. Repeat continuously for the suggested number of repetitions without pausing between jumps. And don't forget to breathe!

FULL SQUAT

The Payoff: Gives your butt a shapely boost and firms your thighs, while increasing flexibility.

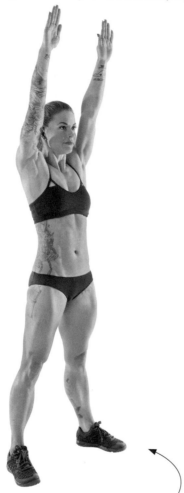

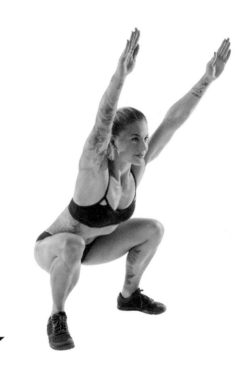

Flex at the hips first, pushing them back and down as the knees bend and spread out, and bringing your arms in front of you. Lower your butt past your knees all while keeping your belly flexed. You should still be rooted in your heels.

Stand straight, with good posture. Pull your navel in toward your spine. Position your feet between hip width and shoulder width. Point your toes out about 15 degrees, not too much. Stay rooted in your heels; you should still be able to lift your toes slightly. Raise your arms overhead, and keep them straight.

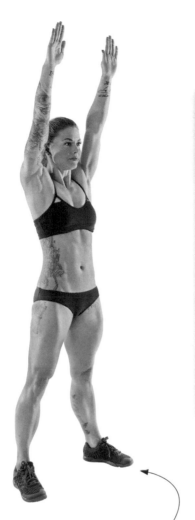

Where It Burns: Butt, hips, hamstrings, and frontal thighs, tummy.

Blunders to Avoid: Don't let your knee extend too far past your toes. It's natural for it to come out further than in a normal squat, but you'll feel less strain if you initiate the movement from your hips instead of shooting your knee forward to start. Don't hunch, lean back, or rock as you squat; this can hurt your back and it won't help you squat any lower.

Tip: If you've never done squats before, position a chair or bench behind you. As you squat down, sit on the seat for just a moment, with your hands straight up in the air. Without rocking forward, stand and come to a fully erect position. Keep your butt tight as you stand tall.

Return to the starting position by standing through your heels and squeezing your glute muscles hard on the way back up. Finish by standing tall and taut. Throughout the squat, always keep your weight on your heels and knees out. Continue squatting for the suggested number of repetitions.

SINGLE-LEG SQUAT

The Payoff: This exercise not only sculpts and tightens your booty and thighs like nobody's business but also indirectly promotes muscle growth across the rest of your body, in places such as your abs, chest, and back. It can also increase endurance in the hamstrings, hips, and thighs, as well as some other leg muscles. This movement is great for balancing your stability.

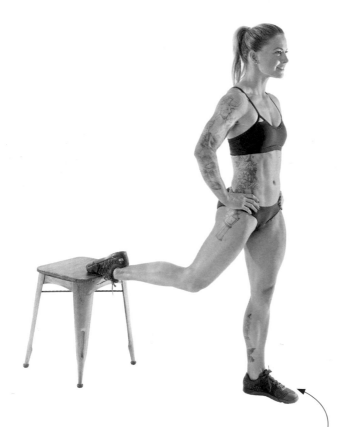

Use a sturdy chair or bench and place it behind you. Take a step away from the bench. Place your back leg on the bench, toe down. Stand straight up, with erect posture.

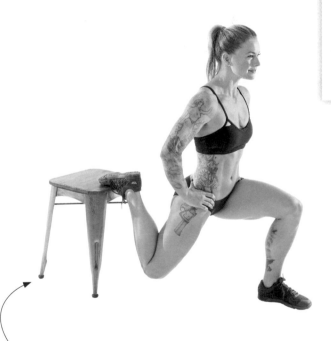

Where It Burns: Glutes, hips, and thighs.

Blunders to Avoid: Your knee should not drift over or past the toe. Also, try not to round your back during this exercise. When your lower back is rounded, you're more susceptible to injuries such as a bulging (herniated) disk.

Tip: If you slow down during the descent, you'll stimulate greater muscle toning and development, particularly in your booty and thighs.

Flex your hip and squat down toward the floor. Hips should go back and down. Try to get your hip crease to come below the top of your knee. Keep your tummy tight. Continue squatting for the suggested number of repetitions.

Better Your Booty with Ass-tounding Exercises   239

THE JUMP SQUAT

The Payoff: Here's a move that gives you the same benefits as standard squats—full-body conditioning, core strength, and stability—plus some extras: balance, coordination, explosive power, and one heck of a cardio burst. Also, this exercise is a great butt lifter, which I love.

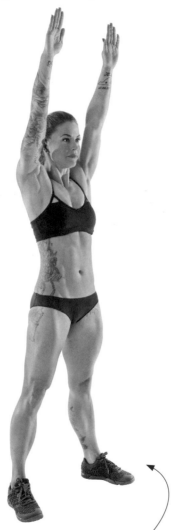

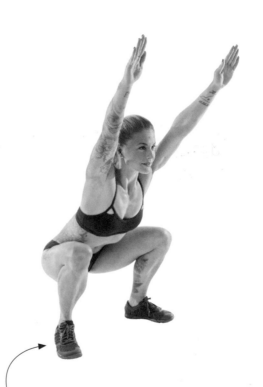

Squat down, pushing your hips back and down, knees out. Be sure to come down to where your hip crease is below the top of the kneecap or thigh.

Stand with your feet slightly wider than shoulder width apart. Keep your tummy tight and raise your arms overhead, just as you would for a squat.

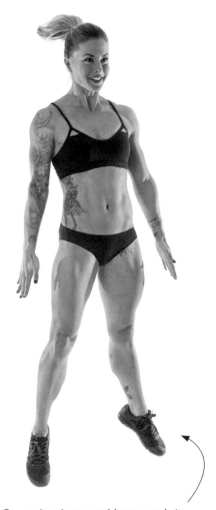

Come back up and jump up into the air as high as you possibly can while sqeezing your butt. Land on your heels softly. You can string these together for best results. Repeat the jump squat for the suggested number of repetitions.

LUNGES

The Payoff: In my opinion, the lunge (also known as the walking lunge) and all variations are the best exercises for the glutes. So for that sexy booty (a booty that looks so good in barely there shorts that men drool when they see it), lunges are a must.

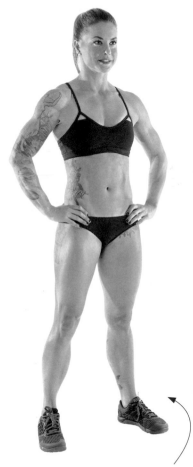

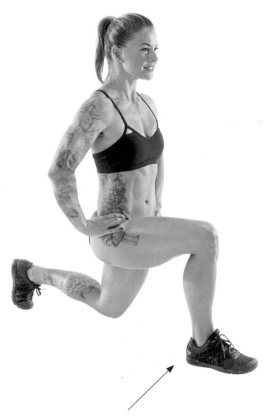

Step forward on your right leg; let your back left knee drop to the floor. Your front knee is bent so that your leg forms a 90-degree angle to the floor and your back leg is angled the same way.

Push up through the back toe while the weight of your body is in the front heel to come back up to a full standing position. Repeat the exercise on the opposite leg. Perform the exercise for the suggested number of repetitions.

Where It Burns: Glutes, hips, thighs, and calves.

Blunders to Avoid: Don't take baby steps as you lunge forward. Little steps place too much stress on the front knee, increasing your chance of a tendon strain. Take a large enough step so that your front heel is nearly two feet in front of your back knee as it flexes down toward the floor. You can feel your weight in the heel, not the toe. To alleviate stress on your knees, don't let your knee to move too far over your toes as you step forward.

Tip: Keep your torso upright through the move, and focus on moving it up and down, not rocking backward and forward. This balances your weight evenly, allowing you to target more muscle. Try not pausing in between lunges for more intense results.

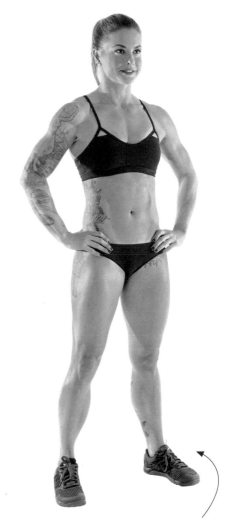

Return to the full standing position.

VARIATIONS OF THE LUNGES

Variation: The Jumping Lunge. Begin by standing straight, with your feet about shoulder width apart and your hands on your waist.

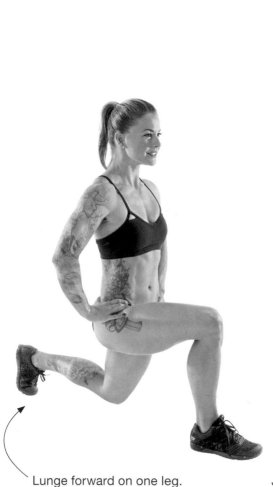

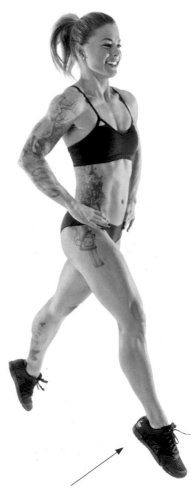

Lunge forward on one leg.

Jump up; switch legs and lunge forward on that opposite leg. Keep your tummy tight the entire time. Continue lunging in this fashion for the suggested number of repetitions. Your knee should "kiss the ground" or hover right above it.

STEP-UPS

The Payoff: When the American Council on Exercise sponsored some research to identify which exercises work the butt best, one of the moves that made the grade was the Step-Up. Add this to your workouts and you'll never stress about a saggy butt again. Also, this exercise is excellent for strengthening your core balance, the thighs, and it puts minimal stress on your knees.

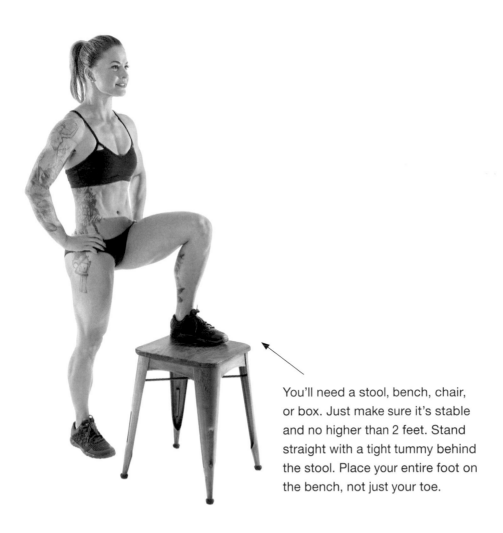

You'll need a stool, bench, chair, or box. Just make sure it's stable and no higher than 2 feet. Stand straight with a tight tummy behind the stool. Place your entire foot on the bench, not just your toe.

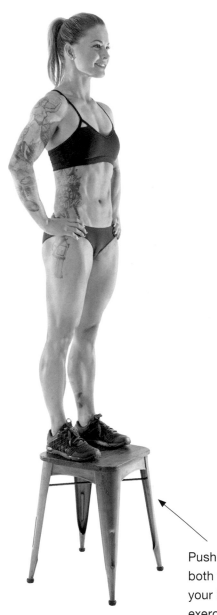

Where It Burns: Hips, glutes, thighs, and tummy.

Blunders to Avoid: Go slowly and resist the desire to rely on momentum; controlled movement is the secret to faster results. Keep a strong back, meaning stand tall during the entire exercise.

Tip: You can gradually increase the difficulty of this exercise by increasing the step height, holding dumbbells in either hand, or increasing the speed of the movement during the exercise.

Push through your heel and step up on the stool with both feet. Step back down to the same side. Alternate your legs each time you step up. Continue the exercise for the suggested number of repetitions.

PUSH-UP

The Payoff: Push-ups build endurance, strength, and muscle.

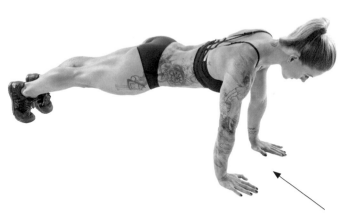

Begin in a plank position, with your feet outstretched behind you, close together, and your hands under your shoulders—not outside your shoulders. Keep your tummy super-tight throughout the movement.

Where It Burns: You may not realize that the push-up affects almost every part of your body—even your fingers and hands. This move targets your biceps, triceps, shoulders and forearms, back, legs, and even your abdominal and glute muscles.

Blunders to Avoid: If you position your hands wider than your shoulders, you'll put strain on the front of your shoulders. As you get into push-up position, make sure your wrists are directly below your shoulders.

Tip: Try to increase the number of push-ups you do on a regular basis, and you'll notice an increase in muscle tone and definition. Push-ups help trigger the release of growth hormone, which helps boost muscle growth.

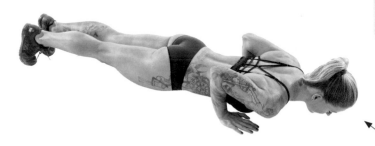

Flex your elbows and pull them towards your rib cage and lower your torso to the floor. Your chest should touch the ground. Then press up with the elbows to lift your body from the floor; lock your elbows at the top of the move while keeping your body taut and in line. Continue the push-up for the suggested number of repetitions.

VARIATIONS OF THE PUSH-UP

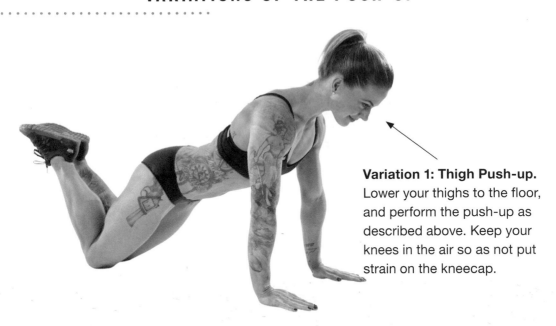

Variation 1: Thigh Push-up. Lower your thighs to the floor, and perform the push-up as described above. Keep your knees in the air so as not put strain on the kneecap.

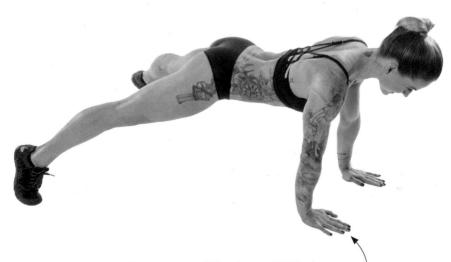

Variation 2: Wide-Legged Push-up. While in the plank position, widen your legs out to the sides, about 2 or more feet. Push up and down as in the standard push-up. Be sure to not let your elbows bow outward during the exercise.

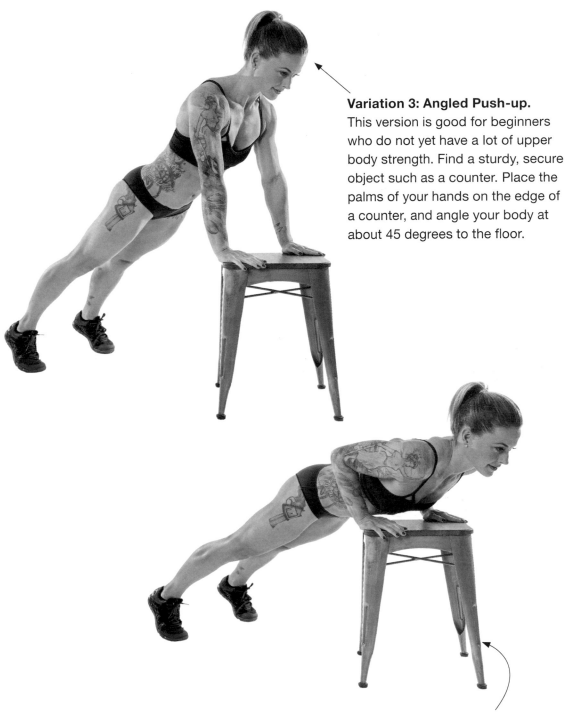

Variation 3: Angled Push-up.
This version is good for beginners who do not yet have a lot of upper body strength. Find a sturdy, secure object such as a counter. Place the palms of your hands on the edge of a counter, and angle your body at about 45 degrees to the floor.

Flex your elbows, lowering your chest to the counter. Push back up to the starting position, locking your elbows.

THE PIKE PUSH-UP

The Payoff: This exercise is great for building shoulder strength. It also strengthens your core and your arm muscles.

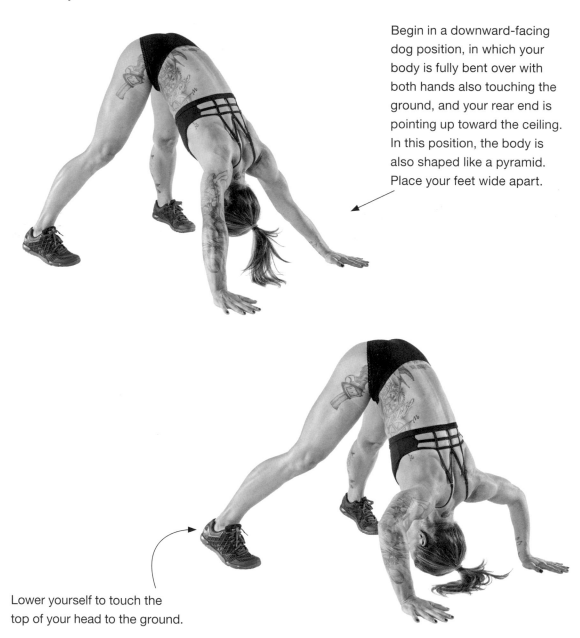

Begin in a downward-facing dog position, in which your body is fully bent over with both hands also touching the ground, and your rear end is pointing up toward the ceiling. In this position, the body is also shaped like a pyramid. Place your feet wide apart.

Lower yourself to touch the top of your head to the ground.

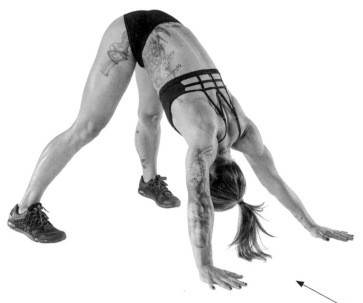

Then push up to return to the start position.

Where It Burns: Your arms, abs, shoulders, back, and chest.

Blunders to Avoid: Don't let gravity do the work for you. The negative, or lowering, portion of the move, builds strength, too.

Tip: If you're just starting out, feel free to limit how far you go down at first. Go halfway down, for example. As your strength builds, you'll be able to touch your head to the ground.

EXPLOSIVE PUSH-UP

The Payoff: The main benefit of doing these push-ups is an increase in strength.

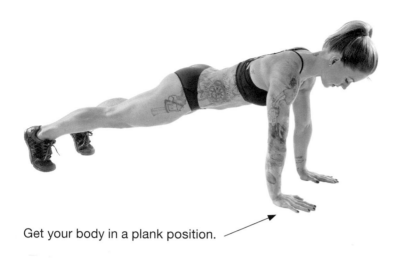

Get your body in a plank position.

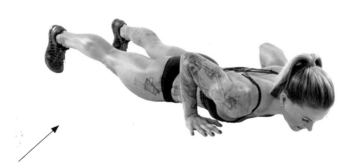

Lower your torso to the floor, keeping a tight belly.

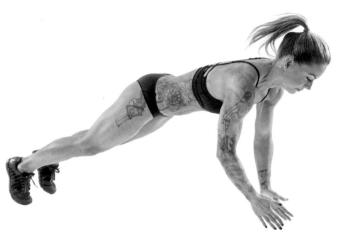

Press back up. But instead of rising up like normal, you explode up. At the top of the move, quickly take your hands off the floor and clap them together in front of you. Return to the plank position and continue the exercise for the suggested number of repetitions. Don't just fall to the ground, catch yourself. Keep it controlled.

Where It Burns: Like the push-up, this exercise works every inch of your body, plus gives you a cardio boost.

Blunders to Avoid: Don't even try this exercise unless you can easily do at least 30 regular push-ups with solid form.

Tip: You can modify this exercise in the same ways that you'd modify a regular push-up: performing it on your knees, for example. Also, if you can't clap (yet), just lift your hands slightly off the floor or go to a thigh push-up version of this.

THE SEXY BACK PUSH-UP

The Payoff: This exercise sculpts your back, shoulders, and chest. That way you can offset wider hips, creating more balanced proportions. It also engages the abs.

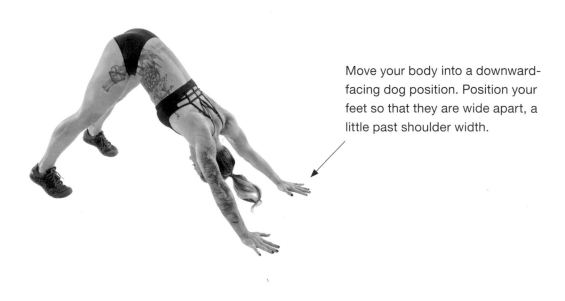

Move your body into a downward-facing dog position. Position your feet so that they are wide apart, a little past shoulder width.

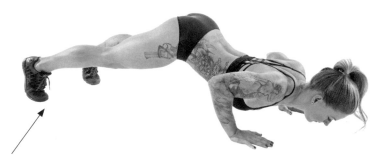

Lower your body, and scoop your chest forward, grazing the floor. Keep your tummy tight; don't drop your hips.

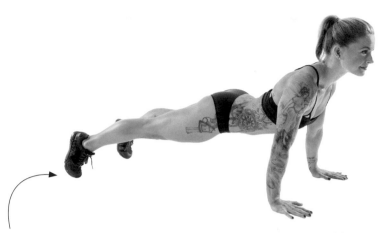

Push all the way up, elbows locked, back to a plank position. Then move back into that downward-facing dog position. Continue the exercise for the suggest number of repetitions. Be sure not to let your hips drop at all.

Where It Burns: Back, shoulders, arms, chest, and abs.

Blunders to Avoid: Don't perform this exercise too fast. The faster you do an exercise, the fewer muscle fibers get stimulated. Your muscles have to be under tension in order to become toned. Performing an exercise slowly and deliberately is best.

Tip: To modify, you can make the scoop a little less dramatic by not grazing the floor as closely.

INCHWORM

The Payoff: This exercise challenges the entire body, plus makes you more flexible. It's called the inchworm because it mimics the forward motion of a worm moving across the ground.

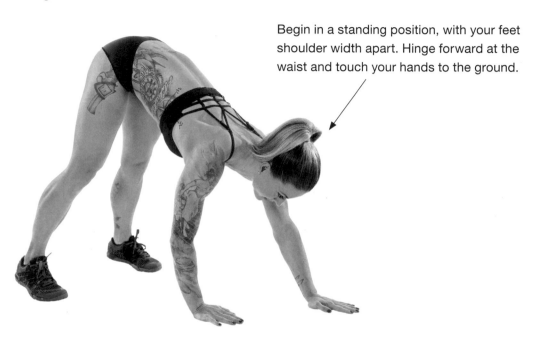

Begin in a standing position, with your feet shoulder width apart. Hinge forward at the waist and touch your hands to the ground.

Walk your hands forward, leaning into your hands. Come to a plank position.

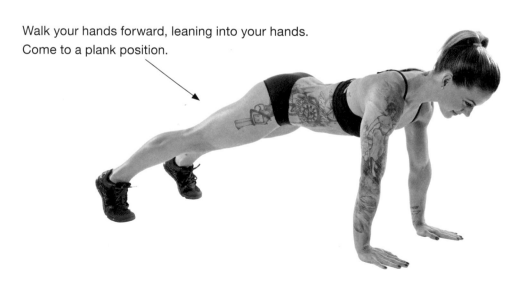

Then perform a push-up.

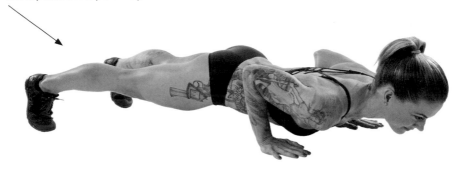

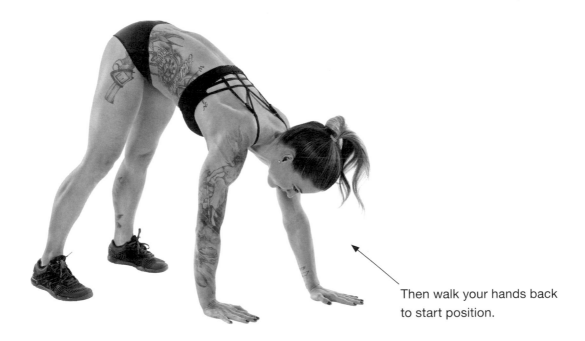

Then walk your hands back
to start position.

Where It Burns: Practically everywhere, but most notably in your arms, hamstrings, and chest.

Blunders to Avoid: To prevent stress on your back during this exercise, keep your back as straight as possible as you perform the move. Don't let your lower back round.

Tip: In order to touch your hands to the floor to begin the exercise, widen your stance. This will allow you to place your hands, palm down, on the floor.

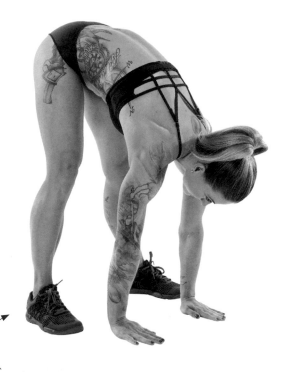

Walk your hands back toward your feet, driving your butt upward and keeping your knees locked. Return to a standing position and repeat the exercise for the suggested number of repetitions.

BURPEES

The Payoff: Burpees basically combine a squat, a push-up, and a vertical leap, and therefore strengthen most muscles of the body, build endurance, and improve sports performance.

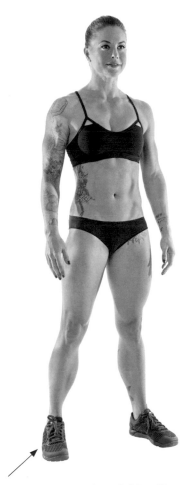

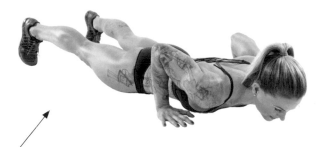

Bend down and place your hands on the ground in front of you. Kick both legs out behind you and lower yourself to the floor.

To begin, stand straight, with your feet a little wider than shoulder width apart and your arms at your sides.

Where It Burns: Everywhere!

Blunders to Avoid: Don't land on the balls of your feet, or you'll fatigue your calves and legs during the jump portion. It puts a lot of pressure on the knees. Always land on your heels. You can step down and up if you have knee issues.

Tip: Keep your tummy tight during burpees in order to prevent stress on your spinal column. Also, don't forget to clap. Not only does this keep you engaged in the exercise, it adds an element of fun to the move.

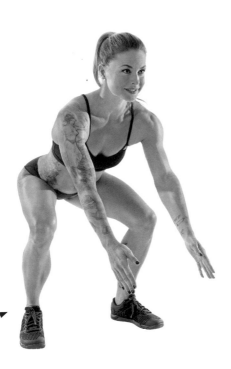

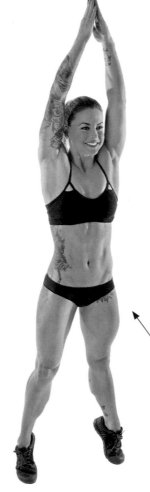

Begin to lift yourself back up from the floor. Jump both legs back up to squat position quickly.

Jump as high into the air as possible from the squat position, reaching both hands above the head. Clap your hands, then land back in the standing position.

VARIATIONS OF THE BURPEES

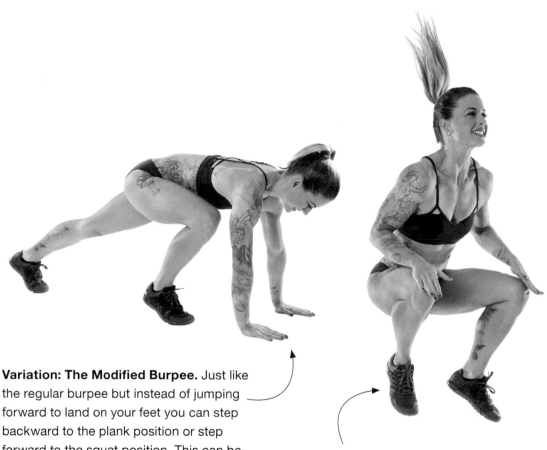

Variation: The Modified Burpee. Just like the regular burpee but instead of jumping forward to land on your feet you can step backward to the plank position or step forward to the squat position. This can be used if the hop is too aggressive for your knees. Do this until you can start jumping instead of stepping.

Variation: The Knee-Slap Burpee. Just like the burpee but you will slap your knees instead of simply jump at the end of the movement. Begin in a squat position with your hands on the ground in front of you. Kick both legs out behind you until you're in a push-up position. Pull both legs back up to squat position quickly. Jump as high into the air as possible from the squat position, reaching both hands above your head. As you jump, bring your knees up to your chest and slap them. Land in standing position.

CRUNCHES

The Payoff: Tight, flat abs, and a strong core for everyday activities.

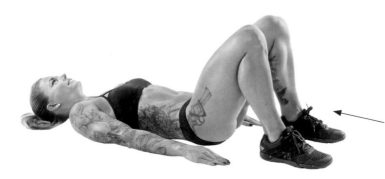

Lie on your back with hands by your side. Your legs should be bent and feet flat on the floor.

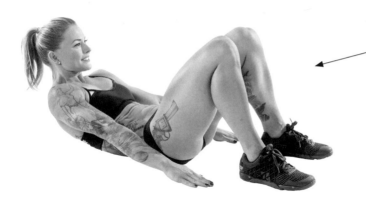

Flex at your tummy so that your back comes all the way up from the floor. Your lumbar area, just above your butt, should stay on the floor. Raise and lower in this fashion for the suggested number of repetitions.

Where It Burns: Abs and core.

Blunders to Avoid: Never use your neck and shoulders to crunch yourself upward. This is painful and not beneficial to the right muscles. When doing crunches, use the strength of your ab muscles to pull your torso up into the crunch position.

Tip: When performing this exercise, keep your lower back pressed down into the floor or exercise mat.

SIT-UPS

The Payoff: The sit-up, when done correctly, tightens and develops the abs. This results in a flatter stomach and the rows of defined abdominal muscles affectionately nicknamed the six-pack.

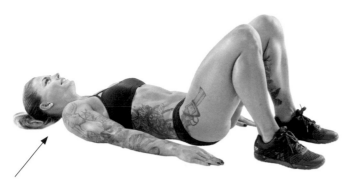

Lie on your back on the floor. Bend your knees and place your legs about a foot apart.

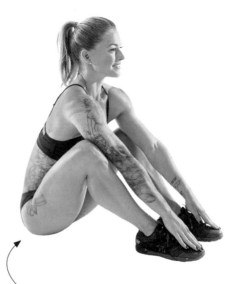

Raise your shoulders and torso off the floor, while holding your arms straight out in front of you for momentum. Come up to a straight-back position (do not slouch forward). Touch your toes. Continue raising and lowering in this manner.

Where It Burns: Abs and core.

Blunders to Avoid: Do not perform sit-ups with your legs straight. Unless your knees are flexed, too much pressure is placed on the base of your spine.

Tip: The more slowly you perform this exercise, the harder you work your ab muscles and the stronger they'll get. If you go fast for more of a cardio burn, make sure you are sitting all the way up.

V-UPS

The Payoff: This exercise firms up abdominal muscles that underlie belly fat and wakes up sluggish circulation so fat burning can proceed. Strong ab muscles burn more calories even at rest and can therefore help prevent your belly bulge from returning.

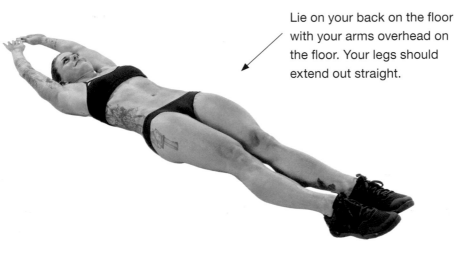

Lie on your back on the floor with your arms overhead on the floor. Your legs should extend out straight.

Bend upward at the waist as you simultaneously lift your legs and arms to meet in a jackknife position. At the peak of this move, you should be balancing only on your bottom. Your legs should be straight at about a 35- to 45-degree angle from the floor.

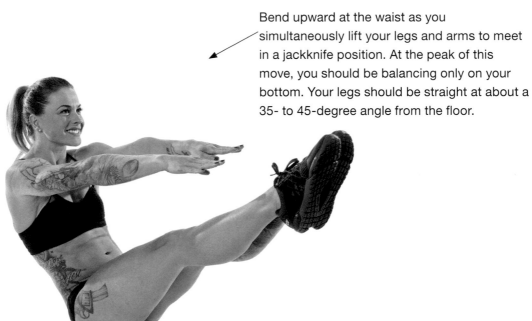

Where It Burns: V-ups primarily target the abs and give you that attractive six-pack. You'll also feel this move in your middle and upper back, as well as in your thighs and hamstrings.

Blunders to Avoid: Don't just do crunches or sit-ups! V-ups offer another way to train your abs and core. Muscles respond to variation; add V-ups to your repertoire. The key is to fully engage your abs and upper back muscles for stability rather than using momentum to propel you through the exercise.

Tip: At the start of this exercise, tighten your stomach muscles, drawing your navel toward your spine. This will stabilize your hips and lower back and strengthen your deepest abdominal muscles.

SINGLE-LEG TOE TOUCHES

The Payoff: This exercise is similar to the V-up and is a great tightener for the upper and lower abdominals.

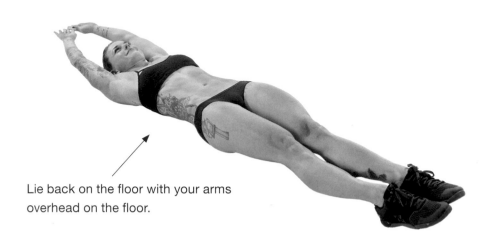

Lie back on the floor with your arms overhead on the floor.

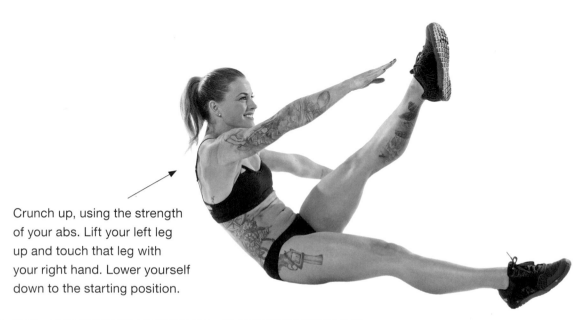

Crunch up, using the strength of your abs. Lift your left leg up and touch that leg with your right hand. Lower yourself down to the starting position.

Return to the start position laying on your back with hands overhead.

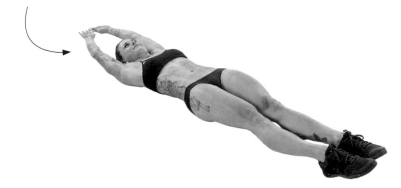

Crunch up again. Lift your right leg up and touch that leg with your left hand. Continue the move, alternating with your left and right legs and hands.

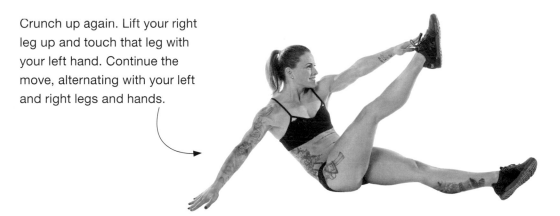

Where It Burns: Abs and core. You'll also feel it in your back, but in a good way.

Blunders to Avoid: Don't tug on your head while doing abdominal exercises or else you'll place unnecessary stress on your neck. This common mistake takes away from the ab-strengthening power of ab work.

Tip: For best results, focus on working your abdominal muscles instead of using your hips to lift your legs up. Keep your back straight as you lower your back and legs toward the ground.

THE BICYCLE

The Payoff: In a study conducted to identify the most effective belly-flattening exercises, researchers at San Diego State University found that one of the best exercises was this bicycle move. So it's a must for your abs!

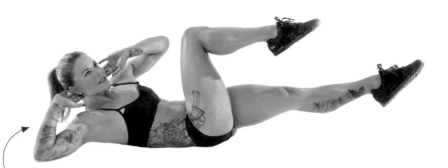

Lie on your back on the floor and keep your lower back pressed as tightly to the floor as you can. Place your hands lightly at the sides of your head, with your fingertips touching your ears. Bend your knees so that they are at about a 45-degree angle to the floor. Lift your shoulders off the floor, bringing one knee to your opposite elbow while straightening out the other leg.

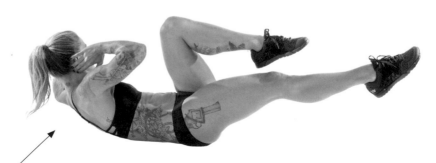

Switch legs and elbows, performing the exercise in an alternating fashion. Continue performing this exercise in a controlled fashion according to the suggested number of repetitions.

Where It Burns: Abs and core.

Blunders to Avoid: You may feel tempted to round your spine and pull on your neck. Doing so takes too much tension off the ab muscles you're trying to work.

Tip: Mentally focus on the muscles you're working during any exercise (abs or otherwise) actually does make a difference in how well you execute the move—and the results you get. Try this on every exercise, and you'll definitely notice a difference.

MOUNTAIN CLIMBERS

The Payoff: This is a great exercise for your core (especially your abs), arms, and legs, and provides a true whole body workout. Plus, this exercise is time-efficient, meaning that it works more muscles in less time. When you do them with all-out effort, mountain climbers are terrific fat burners.

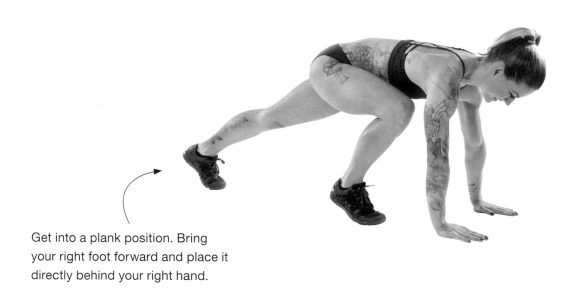

Get into a plank position. Bring your right foot forward and place it directly behind your right hand.

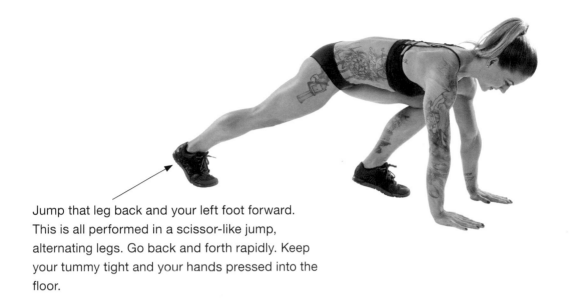

Jump that leg back and your left foot forward. This is all performed in a scissor-like jump, alternating legs. Go back and forth rapidly. Keep your tummy tight and your hands pressed into the floor.

Where It Burns: Everywhere—especially your core!

Blunders to Avoid: Do not bounce up and down. Your upper body should stay stable while your feet move back and forth at a fast pace.

Tip: Keep breathing steadily to help energize the move; try to get into a rhythm.

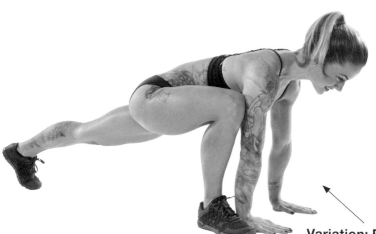

Variation: Power Mountain Climber.
Here's a version that's designed for power: Place the forward foot outside your hand this time.

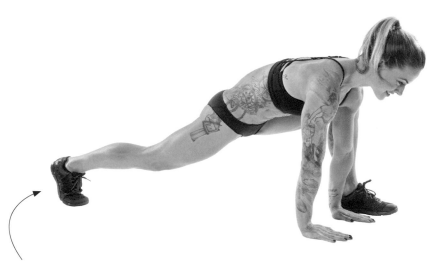

Do scissor-like jumps from this position, alternating legs. Go back and forth rapidly. Keep your tummy tight and your hands pressed into the floor.

BENCH DIPS

The Payoff: This exercise works various muscles simultaneously and will make your body strong, fit, active, and gorgeous.

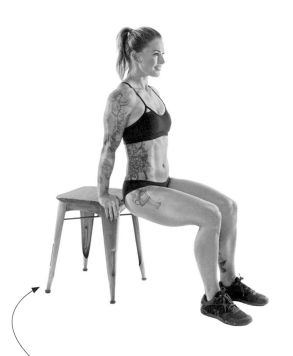

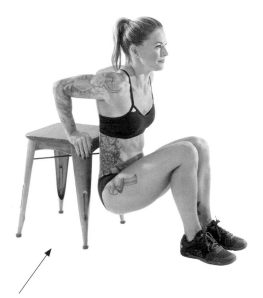

You'll need a stool, bench, chair, or box. Just make sure it's stable. Sit down on the stool. Place your hands on either side of your body, grasping the bench, palms down. Push your hips off the stool, positioning your butt as close to the stool as possible.

Lower your body to the floor. Then press up, locking your elbows to put tension on your triceps at the back of your arms and use your legs to help assist you.

Where It Burns: This move primarily works your triceps but also engages your forearms, shoulders, chest, abs, and lower back.

Blunders to Avoid: Make sure you dip down as far as you can lower yourself. In fact, the lower you go, the better you target the working muscles that are involved in this exercise. Keep your back as close to the object as possible. Don't let your hips pull you away.

Tip: To increase the difficulty, walk your feet out farther to perform the exercise, or elevate one leg as you execute the move.

HAMSTRING ROLLOUT

The Payoff: This exercise is a great way to target the hamstrings, as well as the lower body, abs, and back, to help you stabilize the body.

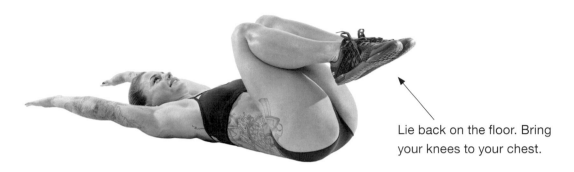

Lie back on the floor. Bring your knees to your chest.

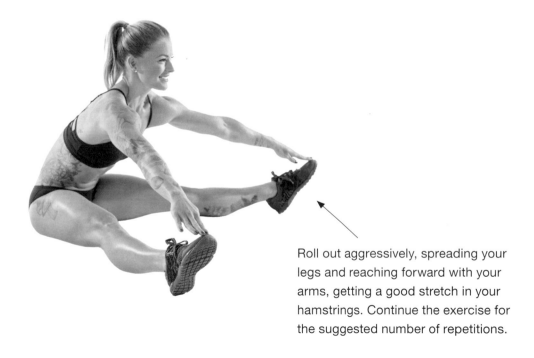

Roll out aggressively, spreading your legs and reaching forward with your arms, getting a good stretch in your hamstrings. Continue the exercise for the suggested number of repetitions.

Where It Burns: Your abs, glutes, and hamstrings.

Blunders to Avoid: Make sure you pause for a quick second between each one, preventing you from rolling right into the next one. You want to start in a paused position and shoot your feet out for the explosiveness.

Tip: Your hamstrings are muscles that are prone to tightness, and it's vital to include this exercise as a part of your regular workouts.

FLOOR WIPERS

The Payoff: Floor wipers combine a leg lift with a trunk rotation. They strengthen the front and sides of your abdomen as well as your hip flexors. A more advanced ab exercise, it's known for its ability to create a nice six-pack.

Lie down on the floor. Place your hands straight out beside you, at shoulder level. Press your palms into the floor to create stability in your core. Lift both legs upward toward the ceiling, so that they're perpendicular to the floor. Keep your feet together.

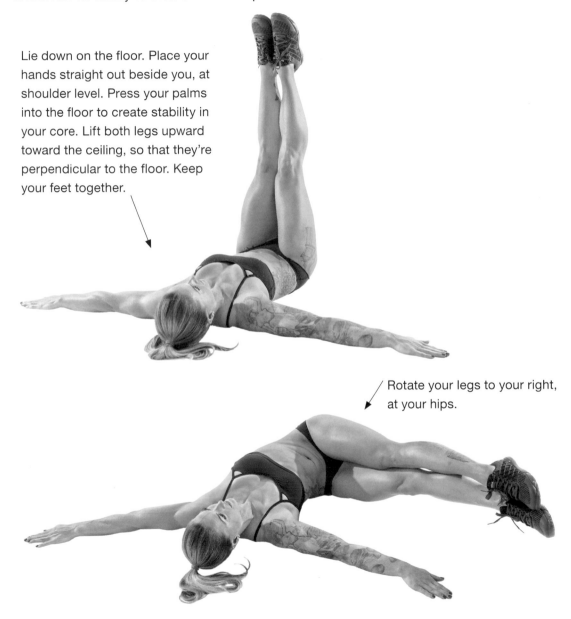

Rotate your legs to your right, at your hips.

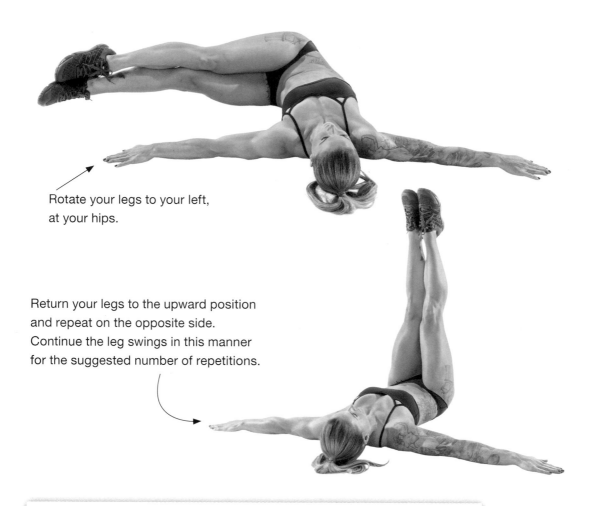

Rotate your legs to your left,
at your hips.

Return your legs to the upward position
and repeat on the opposite side.
Continue the leg swings in this manner
for the suggested number of repetitions.

Where It Burns: Your abs, core, and arms.

Blunders to Avoid: Don't bang your feet on the floor or let momentum take
over the movement. The exercise requires a bit of coordination and balance, as
you are performing both a leg lift and a trunk rotation.

Tip: You can modify this move by not rotating as far on the left or right.
However, try to rotate enough to create tension in your core. To take the
pressure off your lower spine, keep your lower back pressed to the floor and
abdominal muscles contracted throughout the exercise.

SKY HUMPER

The Payoff: This exercise is fun to do and really whips that booty into shape.

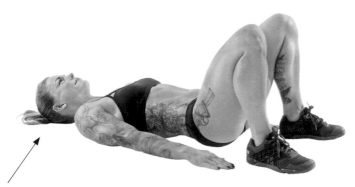

Lie back on the floor. Bend your knees and bring your heels close to your butt. Keep your hands on the floor, palms down.

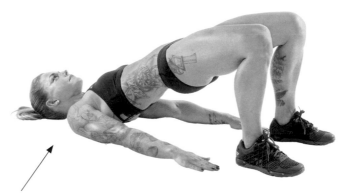

Raise your hips up to create an angled but straight line from your knees to shoulders. Squeeze your glutes, then lower back to start and repeat for the suggested number of repetitions.

Where It Burns: Your glutes, hamstrings, and core. This exercise also engages the erector spinae, a muscle group that spans from the bottom of your neck to your tailbone, as secondary muscles.

Blunders to Avoid: As with most exercises, do not do this one too fast. The movement is small and targeted, so go slow and you will feel your glutes working like crazy.

Tip: To get a greater booty burn, do a single leg move. Lift your butt up toward the ceiling, then take one foot off the floor and straighten the leg toward the ceiling. Repeat the lifting movement with the leg raised. Repeat with the other leg.

Extra Credit: What's the Best Cardio Exercise for Your Booty?

My workouts keep you moving, so you don't have to do any cardio—unless you want to get even more active. If you're in that crowd, please know that any cardio activity that works your ass and thighs does double duty: It will burn fat and tone those areas at the same time.

The following cardio activities will trim and tone your booty, along with my Badass Workout:

Hoof it up a hill. Find a hill in your community and do some walking or running up those hills. Push off your heels as you go. Along those lines, try hiking. With hiking, you're basically doing step-ups on an incline, and we know that those blast your butt.

Do some cycling. Increase the resistance high on a stationary bike and sit toward the back of your seat to fully engage your hamstrings and glutes. Try riding a recumbent bike or a regular one; both are great glute workouts.

Climb stairs. Find a local stadium where you can go up and down the bleachers. Not only will you get an amazing cardio workout but your glutes and thighs will be burning. Or try a stair climber at the gym. Climb at a challenging incline and try not to hold on to the rail.

Go cross-country skiing. This is absolutely the best cardio and toning outdoor workout for your entire body. Or work out on a cross-country ski machine. Both are excellent butt busters, since you are using your glutes and thighs to propel yourself forward.

Get in the pool. Use a kickboard and do as many laps as you can of flutter and butterfly kicks. Your glutes will be screaming.

Sprint for it. Short interval sprints are it! Ever checked out the glutes of a short-distance runner? One glance tells you what running does for your booty. If you want a tighter ass, run on hilly terrain when you train. Sprint up one hill, walk down, and sprint again!

CHAPTER 12

The Badass Workout

THERE'S A DUMB RUMOR out there that in order to get a hot ass, you've got to spend hours sweating the thing off. Au contraire. It's all about doing the right exercises (combined with eating right), and doing them efficiently—and in the previous chapter, I snagged the best ones for you.

The Badass Workout is all about helping you score a firmer butt, but it's also about saving you time. In the beginning, you'll need only a minimum of 12 minutes three times a week. This workout is about training quality, not quantity. Once you progress, you'll spend 20 minutes, and no longer.

These routines may be short, but they're challenging and intense. If you do them correctly, you can bet on three outcomes: 1) Your booty will be shaking by the time you're finished, 2) your whole body will be nicely sore within 24 hours after your workout (that means you did a good workout and your muscles are firming up!), and 3) you'll get gorgeous results. Just follow my easy directions and in 21 days you'll start seeing a tighter, more shapely, cellulite-free booty.

Along the way, you'll also crank up your metabolism, thereby burning more calories all day long, since additional muscle tissue burns up fat stored in your body. For each pound of attractive muscle you put on, your body will automatically incinerate about 30 to 50 extra calories a day.

The Badass Workout is terrific if you're on a budget too. It requires no equipment or pricey gym membership. That's because it uses your own body weight as an exercise tool. Therefore, you can do this workout at home, at your office, in a hotel room—virtually anywhere.

Don't be afraid to hop off your couch and get started. Fitness is a skill, and it has to be learned. If you continue this program with consistency, you will improve, in the same way you learned—and mastered—other skills like typing, riding a bike, or driving a car.

You're the only roadblock standing between you and your full potential and a life that's fun, exciting, and fulfilling. So push your scared, anxious self aside and go forward in this routine with confidence. I know you can do it!

THE THREE LEVELS

I've divided the Badass Workout into three levels, based on your exercise experience and current physical condition:

• **Baby Badass.** This routine is perfect if you're a beginning exerciser, you work out sporadically, or you haven't exercised in a while. It takes only 12 minutes to complete. You'll stay at this level for one month.

• **Certified Badass.** I call this workout an intermediate routine. It's perfect if you've done Baby Badass religiously for a month and are ready to increase your effort or you already exercise but want to try something entirely new, especially for your booty. This routine takes max 20 minutes. You'll stay on it for one month.

• **Royal Badass.** Here's where you really amp it up: an advanced routine to follow if you've done the Certified Badass workout for one month. Feel free to add it to any current workout you're doing. It maxes at 20 minutes.

Across the board, there are 12 distinct workouts. You'll do the first three on Monday, Wednesday, and Friday of the first week; the second three on Monday, Wednesday, and Friday of the second week; the third three on Monday, Wednesday, and Friday of the third week; and the fourth three on Monday, Wednesday, and Friday of the fourth week—for a total of 12 workouts a month.

This system changes up your workouts from week to week—and keeps you motivated because you're not doing the same old workout every week. It also keeps keep your glutes and other muscles guessing. I'm constantly doing new moves and activities for my body. If your workout feels boring in your head, you can bet that the muscles in question are responding with a similar ho-hum. With the Badass Workout, you've got lots of variety, and you'll never get bored with these routines.

I'M A BADASS

Emily, age 22, never really liked working out, probably because she tended to be thin and didn't see the need for exercise. But starting at around age 20, she started gaining fat around her hips and seeing cellulite everywhere on her lower body. Emily definitely had turned into a "skinny-fat" person.

She found my programs through Instagram and figured the short workouts were something she could do. She also decided to try my meal plans and began to follow the Minimalist plan.

After she had followed the program and done the workouts three times a week, the fatty cellulite pockets disappeared—all in less than a month.

Here's what Emily told me: "I was surprised that it worked so well and so fast, because I was always full. I'm loving my new body. I'm not bulky but finally feel firm and toned instead of soft and squishy. My body is hot now!"

Now for Some Guidelines . . .

• Have a physical examination by your doctor before beginning any new program of exercise.

• Follow my directions for the recommended increases in activity. Continue to challenge yourself at each workout to exercise a little harder than you did the previous session. Doing more means more muscle and less body fat.

• Do the exercises in the order given. They're organized into a routine of sets, repetitions, and rounds. A *set* is a group of *repetitions* (the number of times you do a move). A *round* is the entire collection of exercises you do each exercise session. Sometimes I'll ask you to repeat the rounds multiple times. Other times I'll ask you to do the rounds in timed sequences, as rapidly as you can.

• Use only your body weight for these exercises. Just keep moving and keep the pace steady.

• Perform each exercise with good form and pay attention to body positioning. Think about what you're doing and check your form by watching yourself in a mirror if possible.

• Focus intensely on your glutes, tummy, and other muscles while training them. I always feel that you need to feel your butt burn a little bit to trigger and develop noticeable results.

• Don't be afraid to train hard-core. Doing exercises like squats will not make you bulky. This misconception has prevented many women from achieving a sexy fit body and booty.

• Drink plenty of water before, during, and after exercise to prevent your body from becoming dehydrated.

• If you're on the Maintainer or Gainer plan, have a Recovery Shake after your workout.

Here are the Badass Workouts, telling you exactly which exercises to do through the week. Simply follow this schedule and you'll start looking firmer and shapelier in a couple of weeks. The exercises are pictured starting on page 234.

Be sure to record what level and workout you do with your score. You will be able to repeat these workouts at a later date and compare your improvements.

LEVEL 1: BABY BADASS

Week **1**

12 MINUTES MAXIMUM

MONDAY: *Badass Baseline*

Perform one round of this routine.

Jumping Jacks: 50 repetitions
Crunches: 40 repetitions
Squats: 30 repetitions
Push-ups: 20 repetitions
Burpees: 10 repetitions
Jumping Jacks: 50 repetitions

FRIDAY: *Booty Lift*

Perform three rounds of this routine.

Walking Lunges: 10 repetitions on each leg
Inchworms: 7 repetitions
Toe Touches: 10 repetitions on each leg
Squats: 30 repetitions

WEDNESDAY: *Single Jump Jump*

Perform three rounds of this routine.

Step-ups: 20 repetitions
Bench Dips: 15 repetitions
Jump Rope: 100 jumps

MONDAY: *Double Your Fun*

Perform three rounds of this routine.

Set a timer for 12 minutes and try to do all three rounds before it goes off.

Sexy Back Push-ups: 4 repetitions
Jumping Lunges: 8 repetitions on each leg
Sit-ups: 6 repetitions
Jumping Jacks: 20 repetitions

WEDNESDAY: *Let Your Hair Loose*

Timed sequence: Set a timer for 8 minutes and perform the following round as many times as you can before it goes off.

Mountain Climbers: 20 repetitions as fast as you can
Hamstring Rollouts: 7 repetitions as fast as you can
Pike Push Ups: 5 repetitions

FRIDAY: *Get Dirty with It*

Perform five rounds of this routine.

Floor Wipers: 5 repetitions
Push-ups: 7 repetitions
Squats: 15 repetitions

Week
3

MONDAY: *Sweat Like an Animal*

Timed sequence: Set a timer for 6 minutes and perform the following round as many times as you can before it goes off.

Burpees: 5 repetitions as fast as you can
Lunges: 10 repetitions as fast as you can
Squats: 15 repetitions as fast as you can

WEDNESDAY: *Max Your Effort*

Perform three rounds of this routine. Rest one minute between each round.

Round 1:
V-ups: 20 repetitions
Left Single-Leg Squat: 15 repetitions
Right Single-Leg Squat: 15 repetitions

Round 2:
V-ups: 15 repetitions
Left Single-Leg Squat: 10 repetitions
Right Single-Leg Squat: 10 repetitions

FRIDAY: *Beach Body Aspirations*

Perform five rounds of this routine.

Sky Humpers: 10 repetitions
Bench Dips: 10 repetitions
Bicycle: 20 repetitions

Round 3:
V-ups: 20 repetitions
Left Single-Leg Squat: 5 repetitions
Right Single-Leg Squat: 5 repetitions

MONDAY: I Dip, You Dip, We Dip

**Perform five rounds of this routine.
Rest 30 seconds between each round.**

Floor Wipers: 5 repetitions
Bench Dips: 15 repetitions
Lunges: One, hold lunge in the lunge position for 30 seconds. If you have to adjust, the time stops and restarts when you start your lunge again.

WEDNESDAY: Core Basics

Timed sequence: Set a timer for 8 minutes and perform the following round as many times as you can before it goes off.

Hamstring Rollouts: 5 repetitions
Push-ups: 10 repetitions
Sit-ups: 20 repetitions

FRIDAY: Sculpt Me Booty-licious

Timed sequence: Set a timer for 5 minutes and perform the following round as many times as you can before it goes off.

Walking Lunges: 5 repetitions on each leg as fast as you can
Squats: 10 repetitions as fast as you can
V-ups: 5 repetitions as fast as you can

Badass Baseline Reset

The following Monday, repeat the Badass Baseline routine to see if you can beat the number of repetitions you started with. Perform one round of this routine:

Jumping Jacks: 50 repetitions
Crunches: 40 repetitions
Squats: 30 repetitions
Push-ups: 20 repetitions
Burpees: 10 repetitions
Jumping Jacks: 50 repetitions

LEVEL 2: CERTIFIED BADASS

20 MINUTES MAXIMUM

Week
1

MONDAY: *Badass Baseline*

Perform one round of this routine.

Jumping Jacks: 75 repetitions
Sit-ups: 40 repetitions
Squats: 30 repetitions
Push-ups: 20 repetitions
Burpees: 10 repetitions
Jumping Jacks: 75 repetitions

FRIDAY: *Booty Lift*

Perform four rounds of this routine.

Lunges: 5 repetitions on each leg
Inchworms: 10 repetitions
Toe Touches: 10 repetitions on each leg
Jump Squats: 10 repetitions

WEDNESDAY: *Single Jump Jump*

Perform three rounds of this routine.

Step-ups: 15 repetitions
Bench Dips: 15 repetitions
Jump Rope: 50 repetitions
Double-under Jump Rope: 10 repetitions
(A double-under is a jump rope exercise. You
turn the rope for two rotations in one single
jump. So you jump once and while you are in
the air the rope cycles twice instead of just
once like regular jump rope.)

Week
2

MONDAY: *Double Your Fun*

Perform four rounds of this routine.

Set a timer for 16 minutes and try to do all four rounds before it goes off.

Sexy Back Push-ups: 6 repetitions
Jump Squats: 10 repetitions on each side
Sit-ups: 20 repetitions
Jumping Jacks: 40 repetitions

WEDNESDAY: *Let Your Hair Loose*

Timed sequence: Set a timer for 10 minutes and perform the following round as many times as you can before it goes off.

Mountain Climbers: 20 repetitions as fast as you can
Hamstring Rollouts: 7 repetitions as fast as you can
Pike Push-ups: 5 repetitions

FRIDAY: *Get Dirty with It*

Perform five rounds of this routine.

Floor Wipers: 5 repetitions
Clapping Push-ups: 7 repetitions
Jump Squats: 10 repetitions

MONDAY: *Sweat Like an Animal*

Timed sequence: Set a timer for 6 minutes and perform the following round as many times as you can before it goes off.

Burpees: 5 repetitions as fast as you can
Lunges: 10 repetitions as fast as you can
Squats: 15 repetitions as fast as you can

WEDNESDAY: *Max Your Effort*

Perform three rounds of this routine. Rest one minute between each round.

Round 1:
V-ups: 30
Left Single-Leg Squat: 20 repetitions
Right Single-Leg Squat: 20 repetitions

Round 2:
V-ups: 20 repetitions
Left Single-Leg Squat: 15 repetitions
Right Single-Leg Squat: 15 repetitions

FRIDAY: *Beach Body Aspirations*

Perform five rounds of this routine.

Sky Humpers: 10 repetitions
Bench Dips: 12 repetitions
Bicycle: 20 repetitions

Round 3:
V-ups: 10 repetitions
Left Single-Leg Squat: 10 repetitions
Right Single-Leg Squat: 10 repetitions

Week
4

MONDAY: *I Dip, You Dip, We Dip*

**Perform five rounds of this routine.
Rest 30 seconds between each round.**

Floor Wipers: 10 repetitions
Bench Dips: 20 repetitions
Lunges: One, hold lunge in the lunge position for 45 seconds. If you have to adjust, the time stops and restarts when you start your lunge again.

WEDNESDAY: *Core Basics*

Timed sequence: Set a timer for 10 minutes and perform the following round as many times as you can before it goes off.

Hamstring Rollouts: 5 repetitions
Pike Push-ups: 10 repetitions
Sit-ups: 20 repetitions

FRIDAY: *Sculpt Me Booty-licious*

Timed sequence: Set a timer for 5 minutes and perform the following round as many times as you can before it goes off. Rest 2 minutes between each round.

Jumping Lunges: 5 repetitions on each side
Squats: 10 repetitions
V-ups: 5 repetitions

The following Monday, repeat the Badass Baseline routine to see if you can beat the number of repetitions at which you started. Perform one round of this routine:

Jumping Jacks: 75 repetitions
Sit-ups: 40 repetitions
Squats: 30 repetitions
Push-ups: 20 repetitions
Burpees: 10 repetitions
Jumping Jacks: 75 repetitions

LEVEL 3: ROYAL BADASS

Week 1

MONDAY: *Badass Baseline*

Perform one round of this routine.

Jumping Lunges: 30 repetitions
Sit-ups: 40 repetitions
Squats: 30 repetitions
Sexy Back Push-ups: 20 repetitions
Jumping Lunges: 30 repetitions

FRIDAY: *Booty Lift*

Perform five rounds of this routine.

Single-Leg Lunges: 10 repetitions on each leg
Inchworms: 7 repetitions
V-ups: 10 repetitions
Jump Squats: 20 repetitions

WEDNESDAY: *Single Jump Jump*

Perform five rounds of this routine.

Step-ups: 20 repetitions
Bench Dips: 15 repetitions
Double-under Jump Rope: 50 repetitions

MONDAY: *Double Your Fun*

Perform four rounds of this routine.

Set a timer for 16 minutes and try to do all four rounds before it goes off.

Sexy Back Push-ups: 10 repetitions
Jumping Lunges: 16 repetitions on each leg
Sit-ups: 30 repetitions
Jumping Jacks: 30 repetitions

WEDNESDAY: *Let Your Hair Loose*

Timed sequence: Set a timer for 12 minutes and perform the following round as many times as you can before it goes off.

Mountain Climbers: 20 repetitions
Hamstring Rollouts: 7 repetitions
Pike Push-ups: 5 repetitions

FRIDAY: *Get Dirty with It*

Perform seven rounds of the following routine.

Floor Wipers: 5 repetitions
Clapping Push-ups: 7 repetitions
Jump Squats: 10 repetitions

Week
3

MONDAY: *Sweat Like an Animal*

Timed sequence: Set a timer for 10 minutes and perform the following round as many times as you can before it goes off.

Burpees: 5 repetitions
Jumping Lunges: 10 repetitions
Jumping Squats: 15 repetitions

WEDNESDAY: *Max Your Effort*

Perform three rounds of this routine.
Rest one minute between each round.

Round 1:
V-ups: 30 repetitions
Left Single-Leg Squat: 25 repetitions
Right Single-Leg Squat: 25 repetitions

Round 2:
V-ups: 25 repetitions
Left Single-Leg Squat: 20 repetitions
Right Single-Leg Squat: 20 repetitions

FRIDAY: *Beach Body Aspirations*

Perform seven rounds of this routine.

Sky Humpers: 10 repetitions
Bench Dips: 15 repetitions
Bicycle: 30 repetitions

Round 3:
V-ups: 20 repetitions
Left Single-Leg Squat: 15 repetitions
Right Single-Leg Squat: 15 repetitions

MONDAY: *I Dip, You Dip, We Dip*

**Perform five rounds of this routine.
Rest 30 seconds between each round.**

Floor Wipers: 10 repetitions
Bench Dips: 20 repetitions
Lunges: One, hold lunge in the lunge position
for 60 seconds. If you have to adjust, the time
stops and restarts when you start your lunge
again.

WEDNESDAY: *Core Basics*

*Timed sequence: Set a timer for 12 minutes and
perform the following round as many times as you
can before it goes off.*

Hamstring Rollouts: 5 repetitions
Sexy Back Push-ups: 7 repetitions
Sit-ups: 20 repetitions

FRIDAY: *Sculpt Me Booty-licious*

*Timed sequence: Set a timer for 5 minutes and
perform the following round as many times
as you can before it goes off. Rest 1 minute
between each round.*

Jumping Lunges: 6 repetitions on each leg
Jump Squats: 10 repetitions
V-ups: 5 repetitions

Badass Baseline Reset

The following Monday, repeat the Badass Baseline routine to see if you can beat the number of repetitions at which you started. Perform one round of this routine:

Jumping Jacks: 75 repetitions
Sit-ups: 40 repetitions
Squats: 30 repetitions
Push-ups: 20 repetitions
Burpees: 10 repetitions
Jumping Jacks: 75 repetitions

I can just hear you huffing and puffing right now! Remember, though, exercise this intense and fast moving makes you feel good, and when you feel good, you look good. So start imagining how great your booty (and your whole body) is going to look in jeans, shorts, a bikini, and more after you consistently follow the Badass Workout.

PART 4

LIVING THE BADASS LIFESTYLE

CHAPTER 13

Supplements for Success

I TAKE SUPPLEMENTS TO make sure my body is getting all the right nutrients—and to get energized for training and competition.

Food should be the number one source of your nutrition, but I believe that the nutritional value of some foods has decreased, for a bunch of reasons. One is that we're growing food in poor soils that lack nutrients due to overcultivation and misuse of fertilizer and pesticides. Another is that companies are boosting production of vegetables and fruit with fertilizers and chemical additives. Also, far too many of our foods are laced with preservatives, colorings, and other nasty stuff. Science backs me up on this; there have been numerous studies showing that these additives are harming our health, and that many of our foods no longer provide even the minimum nutrition we need on a daily basis to keep us strong and healthy. Case in point, a study published in the *New Phytologist* in 2009 pointed out that the diets of more than two-thirds of the world's population lack many essential minerals, primarily iron, zinc, copper, calcium, magnesium, iodine, and selenium. One of the chief reasons cited by the study for these deficiencies is that our edible crops are grown in mineral-depleted soils.

Our bodies deserve a clean base to work from. If we're loading our systems with chemicals and pollutants, we're hindering the body's ability to create and build healthy cells, including muscle cells. If our nutrition is bad, then our bodies don't have the tools to replace the old cells with healthy new ones. But when our nutrition is good, the new cells are always healthier.

One way to help our cells function optimally is to take supplements in addition to eating clean, healthy food. I realize that supplementation is controversial. Some studies say they work; some studies say they don't. In terms of the Badass plan, I'm often asked, "Will supplements give me a better booty or a more muscular body with less cellulite?" Honestly, I don't know for sure, but I believe that some supplements work toward those ends.

You have to decide for yourself if supplements are right for you. Yes, I believe in supplements, but I'm not advocating that you follow my approach to supplementation. I'm simply providing some information that may help you decide. You have to do what you feel is right for you.

Here's a list of my "don't leave home without" supplements.

ZINC

I take extra zinc because it's an important mineral for active people. In fact, zinc deficiencies are fairly common in athletes who train really hard, especially if they're dieting, too. Exercisers and athletes need additional zinc daily to prevent shortfalls, because the body has no means of storing this mineral.

Zinc is involved in numerous aspects of metabolism. It's required for the production and activity of more than 100 enzymes, and it's involved in boosting immunity, helping the body build new proteins, healing wounds and injuries, and promoting cell division. Zinc is an essential nutritional building block of muscle-building testosterone too.

A short supply of zinc not only messes with testosterone and muscular development. It can also decelerate your metabolism by interfering with the production of thyroid hormones that help regulate metabolism, our bodies' food-to-fuel process. A subpar metabolism makes it much harder to get rid of body fat, and much easier to put it on.

I read a 2003 study that looked at metabolism in men and women who followed a low-zinc diet initially and afterward started supplementing with zinc (about 25 milligrams a day). The low-zinc diet caused drops in metabolism, but about three weeks of zinc supplementation jacked it up again. In fact, the subjects' metabolisms were so high that they started automatically burning around 300 extra calories a day.

I take 50 milligrams of chelated zinc in the morning to ensure myself against a metabolic slowdown. The chelated form of this mineral is very well absorbed by the body.

MAGNESIUM

Intense exercise can deplete your magnesium stores, and magnesium is another mineral involved in metabolism. It's also key for muscle functioning. When you're trying to tighten and tone your body and booty, you certainly don't want a sluggish metabolism or problems moving your muscles.

Magnesium is involved in hundreds of other biochemical reactions in the body. Like zinc, it helps the body create new muscle. It assists in strengthening bone. And it's a heart-friendly supplement because it helps regulate blood pressure.

More recently, magnesium has been proven to help with the problem of insulin resistance. This occurs in the body when cells become insensitive to insulin, which ushers blood sugar into muscle and brain cells for fuel and nourishment. With insulin resistance, sugar has nowhere to go, so it accumulates in the blood, wreaking all sorts of metabolic havoc. Some of that sugar heads to the liver, where it's usually turned right into fat, which ends up padding your booty, abs, and the rest of your body. But with magnesium on the case, you have an indirect fat burner.

Magnesium also helps with a number of other issues:

Headaches and migraines. Magnesium relieves muscle spasms and tension that lead to head and neck pain. It's a great natural remedy for these annoying and often persistent problems.

Insomnia. In addition to unkinking tense muscles, magnesium helps your body produce the sleep hormone melatonin—which means you will sleep better, night after night.

Constipation. Magnesium eases this problem by pulling additional water into your colon and improving muscle function. The "end" result is that your poop train will run more frequently and on time. If you have other digestive issues (including irritable bowel syndrome or Crohn's disease), magnesium supplements may help you.

I take 100 milligrams of chelated magnesium at night prior to bedtime.

Hip Advice: Preworkout Supplements

There's a relatively new category of fitness supplements on the market known as preworkout supplements, promoted as a way to boost your energy while working out. I'm not a big fan of these products. They're typically loaded with sugar, caffeine, and other stimulants, none of which delivers any real nutrition to muscle fibers.

Preworkout supplements may also contain pro-hormones, which are designed to increase the body's natural hormone levels. This is totally inappropriate for a young, growing body. Even for a woman going through menopause, management of hormone levels should be done in a medical setting in conjunction with laboratory testing to ensure that targeted blood levels are achieved and maintained.

My advice to you is not to rely on these supplements. Learn what your own body can do naturally in workouts without relying on artificial and supplemental uppers. I've seen some people become dependent on these products the same way they get hooked on sugar. Bottom line: Put these supplements back on the shelf.

BRANCHED CHAIN AMINO ACIDS (BCAAS)

I love this protein supplement, which typically comes in capsule form. It can't be beat for improved recovery after workouts, reduction of muscle soreness, and greater energy during long workouts. Plus, it just may be a fat burner. Read on!

For background, BCAAs are a family of three amino acids (pieces of protein) that includes leucine, isoleucine, and valine. Structurally, each BCAA has a shape that resembles a tree branch, which is why these aminos are named "branched-chain." The BCAAs are all essential amino acids, meaning you have to get them from the food you eat. Cells use them to create protein, including muscle protein.

BCAAs are metabolized differently from all other amino acids. They bypass your liver and are metabolized directly in your muscle tissue, meaning that they more directly fuel the muscle-building process.

Getting these amino acids to your muscles after a workout helps muscles grow and develop—a benefit that has been well documented in research. In one study, athletes took BCAA supplements, or a placebo, over an experimental period of 21 days. By the end of the trial, they had increased their lean mass by 1.5 percent and better maintained the size of their arms and legs. Plus, their leg strength increased, as compared to those taking a placebo.

Best of all, it looks like BCAAs just might help the body burn fat. This is good news if you're among the women who seem to find it harder than others do to lose those stubborn pounds. One strategy might be to use BCAAs to complement the Badass plan.

There's some pretty good science out there to support this strategy. A study of wrestlers showed that those who supplemented with BCAAs, in addition to following a reduced-calorie diet, lost more weight and body fat (especially in the belly) than those in a control group who didn't supplement or diet.

Okay, BCAAs seem to work for wrestlers, but what about us women?

Again, the news looks promising. A study out of the journal *Age* showed that a dose of

12 grams of leucine in combination with some good fats—oleic acid and DHA (found in fish oil)—resulted in a close to 4-pound weight loss within two weeks in women over age 38. The researchers chose the BCAA leucine because of its effects on fat loss in other studies.

Of course, more research is needed, but these studies make a pretty solid case for BCAA supplements when you want to burn a little extra fat.

BCAAs work best when you stay active. I take mine before my workouts and or after. After I started adding BCAAs to my supplement program, I did notice a difference. I had more energy in my workout and I improved my body composition.

I'M A BADASS

Meet Maria, age 52. She's a yoga enthusiast and a marathon runner who was looking to firm and shape up her body a little more. She felt that because she was in her fifties, her body wasn't responding as quickly as it had in her youth. She'd been on other diets but was never able to stick to them long-term.

Maria did the plan with full force. She followed the diet, she took a number of the supplements I talk about here, and she added my exercises to her already active routine.

Maria told me: "I love this program because I never feel hungry. It provides a lot more food than I imagined. As for my training, I had always carb-loaded before any major run. This time, I added a few bricks instead and immediately felt the difference. Before long, I was running marathons in less time than before. This plan worked wonders for me. My body changed and I looked fitter, not leaner or bigger but stronger and more toned. I told my daughter about it and we're both on the program now."

FISH OIL SUPPLEMENTS

I take these because there's just so much research out there that supports their benefit, I feel it would be foolish not to. Fish oil, of course, comes from fish, a supersource for omega-3 fatty acids, which are vital for brain and heart health. They also work as natural anti-inflammatories, and thus are a great treatment for sports injuries or aching joints.

There's a fat-burning benefit from fish oil supplements too, especially if you're an exerciser. In a 2007 study published in the *American Journal of Clinical Nutrition*, Australian researchers looked into the benefits of fish oil and exercise, alone or in combination, on body composition and cardiovascular health. Approximately 80 overweight men and women participated and were randomly assigned to one of four groups. They blindly took either 6 grams of fish oil a day or 6 grams placebo (sunflower) oil. Within each oil treatment group, some were also instructed to exercise three times a week. The study continued for three months.

The results of the study were impressive. Both the fish oil and exercise independently reduced body fat. Plus, supplementation improved the volunteers' heart health: it lowered triglycerides, increased the good HDL cholesterol, and improved the pumping action of the heart.

So, to possibly improve your heart health and alter your body composition, consider becoming an Omega Woman: Get more omega-3s through diet and supplements. There are two kinds of omega-3s found in fish oil: DHA and EPA, which are responsible for the benefits of fish oil. Only 25 percent of us get *any* DHA or EPA in our diets on any given day.

You want a high-EPA fish oil! The higher ratio of EPA to DHA provides all the inflammation reduction and recovery benefits you expect from a high-quality fish oil while avoiding the body fat increases associated with excessive intake of DHA. Look for brands that carry 750 mg of EPA per dose.

Even though I might eat a couple of servings of omega-3-rich fish a week, I still pop 1 to 3 grams of fish oil daily, with emphasis on the EPA.

SUPPLEMENTATION IS ONE OF the easiest moves you can make, and takes only seconds a day. Added to a nutrient-rich diet and a consistent workout program, supplements can help you boost your health, and quite possibly assist your body in fat burning and muscle building. Supplements are definitely worth considering in your quest to become a Badass.

CHAPTER 14

Living the Plan

IF YOU'RE LIKE MOST of the people I work with, believing in and following the Badass plan has changed you inside and out. I love hearing from women who tell me that they've lost pounds and inches, reshaped their bodies, and gotten tighter, sexier booties. And not only has the Badass plan strengthened their bodies, it has strengthened their spirits. Women become more confident, more focused, and brimming with greater self-love.

When you first start out on a program, usually the experiences and initial successes are new, fresh, and exciting. The question is: How do you keep it going year after year after year? Another way to ask it: How do you continue to live the Badass lifestyle for a lifetime?

There are countless ways to do this, and I'll share my suggestions with you here.

THE BADASS PLAN ALLOWS "CHEATS"

Once you've stayed on one of the Badass plans for 21 days, you can "cheat," but only if you want to. Let me define what I mean by "cheat," and how to do it without blowing the whole plan.

When I say "cheat," I'm talking about an individual meal or snack, not a whole day or week of cheating. A cheat meal is simply one where you add a food to your plan that you might not otherwise eat. You can cheat on the Minimalist or Modifier plans, for instance, by eating a carb that's not a primo carb, perhaps at dinner. That "cheat" carb might be some pasta or a baked potato. Or you might add a slice of pie to your Badass meal.

Schedule your cheat and stick to it. If you don't want it and don't use it, you lose it. Basically, if you're going to cheat, stick to *planned cheating*—periodically going off the plan and permitting yourself to eat foods that typically are not thought as "plan" or "primo" foods (such as pizza, ice cream, fries, desserts, and so forth). In some ways, this strategy isn't really "cheating" per se, because you're scheduling it, but I stick with that word because people can relate to it, and the idea of being able to cheat gives people a little psychological boost.

You have to be careful with cheat meals, though. They can turn into cheat days that turn into cheat weeks, and before long, your favorite all-you-can-eat buffet restaurant will be sending you flowers and coupons. That's why I don't recommend cheat meals more than once a week at the most. Give me a couple of cheat meals a month, and I'm completely happy. I believe in real-world dieting; I just want the option to eat what I want—occasionally.

Cheat meals don't even have to be junk food; they can include any food that's not in the primo category. Personally, I don't even like junk food. Clean eating does that to you; the more you eat clean, the less junk you want to put in your body. I feel like crap if I eat too much junk.

Here's how I cheat. On Friday for a snack, I might treat myself to a cupcake, but only if I plan to have it. On a Sunday, if I go out for brunch with my girlfriends, I order scrambled eggs and veggies; then we all split an order of French toast for the cheat. (I spread mine with peanut butter to balance out my protein, carbs, and fat.) The entire brunch is a heavenly scenario that gives me freedom, dietary leeway, and enjoyment of a meal with friends.

When you decide on your cheat meal, make it worth it—something you really enjoy and can eat without guilt.

I put a couple of other stipulations on cheat meals: First, don't eat a cheat portion so large that you stuff yourself to the point of discomfort. Eat until you're satisfied, but that's it. If you're leaving the table saying "I'm stuffed," or if you're feeling sick, or if you have to lie down because you overdid it, that's when you know you messed up and blew the plan.

Second, if you suffer from binge eating or another eating disorder, cheat meals may not yet work for you until you've got your condition cured or under control. This is because cheat meals can lead to binges in susceptible people. But that's usually a very small minority of dieters. Ninety-nine percent of people are ready and motivated to hit the plan hard after a cheat meal.

THE BADASS PLAN IS AN "ANYWHERE" PROGRAM

Quite often, the downfall of any diet or workout program is dining out or traveling. People tend to throw in the towel in these situations and use them as excuses to overeat or not exercise.

Not with the Badass plan—you can take it anywhere and do it anywhere. If you're someone who eats out often at restaurants, have no fear. You've got the green light to eat at just about any type of restaurant on the planet; just make healthy choices. Those include: grilled meats, poultry, or fish; grilled vegetables such as broccoli or green beans; salads with dressing on the side; baked potatoes or sweet potatoes; and small portions of rice or pasta (no bigger than a handful). Make those sorts of selections and you've just ordered a great Badass plate.

Some other tips:

• Just say no to the bread bowl. Ask the waitstaff not to serve you bread, or if they come to your table with it, politely ask them to take it away.

• Be inquisitive about your meal. Ask the server: How many ounces are in the salmon? How is it cooked? How large are the servings?

• Ask for substitutions. For example, replace mashed potatoes with mixed veggies or the veggie of the day. Don't want any starches? Order a double portion of veggies instead of the usual combo of one veggie and one starch.

• Be sure to have a fat of some sort with your protein and carbohydrate. Most places will have avocado or guacamole; ask to add it on. You need the fat to help prevent overeating.

• Stay off the booze. At restaurants, I order my "Pretend and Tonic." That's a glass of club soda on the rocks with a wedge of lime. It looks like I'm having a cocktail, but I'm really not. (At home, you'll find yourself not needing to decompress with that nightly glass of wine. On the Badass plan, you'll feel so much more even-tempered and patient that you won't desire any sort of alcoholic beverage.)

• Avoid cream soups or cream anything! Soups are fine if they're broth based, but many soups have cream in them to help make them be more filling.

HAVE BADASS, WILL TRAVEL

I'm on the road several months out of a year, so I know how challenging it can be to stick with your plan while traveling. But it's completely doable. Some strategies I've found to be helpful:

• Invest in a good lunchbox or cooler and some good containers. Smaller containers are generally better so you can have a nice snack without pulling out the fridge from your cooler. I like to use 1- to 1½-cup sizes, for ease of keeping food items separate.

• Prepack your meals. Yep, during your meal prep for the week, go ahead and prepack your travel meals. If you can premeasure and layer one meal in one container, that's ideal. For example, try sweet potato hash on the bottom and rotisserie chicken on top for 2 bricks. I bring an avocado with me, or single packets of peanut butter. (Note for fliers: The TSA doesn't allow peanut butter in a package over 3 ounces to pass through security. I've tried it and failed! So you have to carry little packets of peanut butter and let them go through security with all liquid toiletries.) Foods that travel well include hard-boiled eggs, deli meat (turkey or ham), apples, individual-size containers of applesauce, grapes, avocados, and individual packets of butter.

• Look for "plan" foods on the go. Use my dining tips strategies above to order foods that work with the plan. If you're grabbing a sandwich on the go (at an airport, for example), request that it be lettuce-wrapped (no bun). At home, choose a sandwich made with flatbread or pita bread; these are typically healthier. Ask for double meat, too, for some extra appetite-curbing protein. Also, try eating half the sandwich and saving the rest for later, especially if you find yourself in an emergency situation where there's no food around and you're ravenous.

• Drink plenty of water while on the road. Flying is dehydrating, and drinking enough water will prevent that. Water also fills you up and keeps you from getting too hungry.

• Do your Badass workout. My exercises are mostly body weight moves, which means they can be done anywhere, anytime. Clear some space in your hotel room and get moving! Working out while on the road will keep you mentally and physically energized, focused, and alert. Plus, you're less likely to gain any travel or vacation weight on the trip.

I'M A BADASS

Rachel, age 36, is always on the go. She flies nearly every week for business and has little to no time to cook meals at home. She works out when she can, but isn't consistent.

A friend told Rachel that my plan was "anywhere friendly," so she decided to put it to the test.

"Once I learned how to prep my meals for traveling, it was easy—almost too easy! While eating out, I knew I had to choose a protein, carbohydrate, and fat—so designing a menu while on the road was simple," Rachel said.

"Initially, I just wanted to learn how to eat healthfully while traveling. But I came away with so much more. My body shape changed and became leaner. My energy was up. I was never hungry. My sex drive went through the roof to the point that my husband and I are now expecting our first child. I love this plan."

RECRUIT A BUDDY

They're better together—exercise and healthy eating, that is. Do the Badass plan with a buddy, neighbor, family member, partner—anyone who's motivated to do it and has a schedule similar enough to yours that you can get together regularly and support each other.

Having a buddy—for the diet, the workout, or both—can lead to better results. A lot of research has shown that people are very successful when using a buddy system while getting in shape. If you schedule workout times, you're less likely to back out if you know you'll be letting someone else down. When one of you feels like vegging on the couch, the other partner can motivate you to head to the gym or stick to the plan. That's the power of accountability.

Make the partnership fun, too. Be competitive, for example, if that's your thing. One good way to keep each other fired up is to stage a fitness challenge to see who can do the most reps or rounds. Maybe the loser has to buy a can of protein powder for the winner or pay the winner five bucks.

Share inspirational quotes or recipes with each other. Go to restaurants together and help each other select healthy menu items. If one of you has a "down" day and wants to slack off, the other should be there for encouragement to pick you up and keep you going.

Involve your whole family, including your kids. Family mealtime is a great opportunity to improve your family's diet and help get everyone to a healthier place in life. Studies show that family meals help people better control their portions, eat more nutritious meals, and strengthen the family bond. Along those lines, start promoting family activities, such as bike rides, swimming, hiking, camping, skiing, and other sports.

What evolves is a support group for each family member. If the shared plan encourages better eating and more physical activity, each member is more likely to stay engaged. These shared moments can instill healthy habits in your family for years to come.

Hip Advice: Do It with Your Guy

More and more, guys are watching their weight and paying as much attention to nutrition as we do. If your guy needs to lop off a few (or more) pounds, he can do it easily on the Badass plan. You can both eat the same food—no need to prepare a second meal for him—but with a difference. Your guy will eat more bricks at his meals.

THE MODIFIER PLAN FOR GUYS

A guy between 5′6″ and 5′9″ eats between 11 and 15 bricks a day.
A guy between 5′10″ and 5′11″ eats between 14 and 21 bricks a day.
A guy 6′ or taller eats between 16 and 25 bricks a day.

THE MAINTAINER PLAN FOR GUYS

A guy between 5′6″ and 5′9″ eats between 13 and 18 bricks a day.
A guy between 5′10″ and 5′11″ eats between 15 and 22 bricks a day.
A guy 6′ or taller eats between 17 and 26 bricks a day.

THE GAINER PLAN FOR GUYS

A guy between 5′6″ and 5′9″ eats between 14 and 19 bricks a day.
A guy between 5′10″ and 5′11″ eats between 16 and 21 bricks a day.
A guy 6′ or taller eats between 21 and 28 bricks a day.

What about the Minimalist plan for guys? That's easy: When serving up his plate at meals, give him between 25 and 50 percent more food that you put on your plate.

WORK ON REWARD

I'm a huge fan of rewarding yourself for success with diet and exercise, and here's why. The challenge with changing to a healthier diet and a more active lifestyle is that the fitness rewards don't come fast enough for most of us. We need short-term rewards to keep us going. There's no better way to fuel motivation than immediate gratification.

If you've stuck with it, even for a week, treat yourself to something you've wanted, like that handbag, new running shorts, a visit to a day spa, or some other non-food-related reward that you can enjoy *now*. Whatever your rewards are, keep them in sight and focus on the prize. And guilt free!

BANISH STRESS EATING

One of the big derailing factors I see happen to a lot in people is stress. Mental and emotional overload have a way of sending us straight back into fattening snack or couch mode. Here's some good news: By learning better ways to react when you're stressed, you can stop any weight gain that's caused by emotional eating and stay on the healthy straight and narrow.

• Get moving to ease stress. Exercise churns out feel-good endorphins that neutralize stress, along the way making you feel better physically and emotionally and helping you burn fat. Another technique that can mediate stress eating is yoga, one of my favorite activities. It's known to lower stress so that you aren't always diving into a gallon of ice cream for relief. Yoga has a world of other benefits too, such as strength, flexibility, and antiaging.

• Identify whether you're truly hungry or desiring to eat for emotional reasons. When you're tempted to binge, ask yourself why. Are you truly hungry or simply super stressed out? If it's stress doing the tempting, find another activity such as exercise, taking a walk, calling a friend, or going to a movie to take your mind off things.

• Eat on a regular schedule. This means having your meals and snacks at fairly fixed times. Doing so can help you break the habit of impulse eating. Don't skip meals to save calories, either. This can lead to hunger later in the day, and the temptation to overeat.

• Avoid temptation. Remove all high-calorie junk foods from your kitchen. When unhealthy food is out of sight, it's out of mind.

• Rearrange your life. Consider whether you might be overcommitted on your job and in your day-to-day activities. Try to put more balance in your life so that you have time for pleasure, relaxation, and spiritual fulfillment—all life choices that will counteract the negative effects of stress.

• Get enough rest. If you're really stressed out, get more rest, take naps, and have a good night's sleep. During rest (including sleep), your body is actually very busy. It works on healing injuries and infections. It flushes your body of toxins and waste products. It replenishes fuel in your muscles. And it dissipates stress.

• Talk it out. You may just want to pour your heart out to a friend. Just talking to someone you trust can make you feel much better. Seek help from a mental health counselor if your stress won't let up, or you can't control your eating by yourself.

MAINTAIN A TRUE BADASS ATTITUDE

I'm not talking about about being mean or nasty—far from it. Let me elaborate. We've talked a lot about booty in this book, but now I want to talk about another kind of booty—the one that is defined as treasure.

Our bodies hold the treasure of life inside of them, life that we have been given. Our bodies are good and should be treated with honor every day that we are alive. To do that, I believe you have to focus on five key habits. They're simple things, but they're incredibly powerful. If you work at them daily, they can change the precious treasure that is your life. Like anything, it just takes some practice and some belief. Here they are:

1. SET BIG GOALS, THEN BREAK THEM DOWN.

I never aim low. If you want to achieve big things in this life, I believe you have to set major long-term goals that push your limits and really stretch your abilities. Running a 5K might be your big goal right now, or maybe it's to add 50 pounds to your squat. It doesn't matter. Set the bar high, then break it down into small, attainable goals that you can work on every day. Don't focus on the end result. Great long runs begin with mastery of single foot strikes. If you want to squat big, it starts by adding just a few pounds. If you want to lose 20 pounds, it starts with a few lost pounds each week and healthy eating a day at a time. Take these small steps, relentlessly, one foot in front of the other, every day, and your goal will be within reach before you know it.

2. ALWAYS TRY NEW THINGS.

I'm sure you're familiar with the maxim "If you keep doing what you've always done, you'll keep getting what you've always gotten." It makes perfect sense; why do so many people keep expecting their life or body to change when they're so resistant to new experiences and experiments?

Make a habit out of saying yes more often, no matter how anxious, frightened, or resistant you might feel at first. You'll discover that sometimes the things you didn't believe you would enjoy become some of your new favorite activities. You'll never know unless you try.

I used to be afraid to try new things because I feared I would fail. I figured that if I didn't try anything, then I could never fail.

How wrong I was. Had I not tried CrossFit, I would have stayed in bad shape and in a life rut, physically and mentally. Had I not tried NASCAR, you probably never would have heard of me.

It's okay to let yourself fail too. We learn more from failing than we do from succeeding. As Thomas Edison said, "I have not failed. I've just found 10,000 ways that won't work."

There's no failure—except in not trying.

3. DO GOOD WITHOUT EXPECTING ANYTHING IN RETURN.

I'm talking about the "smile stuff." Open the door for someone, smile as they pass by (for no reason other than to pass on a smile), or tell a sales associate's manager how nice an employee was to you. When you start a project or a venture, don't think about the money you could make from it. Instead, focus on maximizing the value you can provide to other people.

Selfless acts like these are highly rewarding. So give more often. The more you do it, the more you'll focus on what matters most: the effort, the daily work, and the additional opportunities for good that it all creates. You'll see, you'll start reaching the big goals more often the more good that you do. It's simple and extremely rewarding.

Always act with the purest of motives, and never expect great things to come your way because you did something good. Do good just for the sake of doing good.

4. LEARN TO PUT YOURSELF FIRST, SOMETIMES.

You have to give to others, but there must be limits. Too much giving without regard to your health can drain you, and that's not good for anyone in your life, especially you.

Be selfish with some of your time. You don't have to go missing in action; just make sure to schedule personal hours on your calendar to read or enjoy a new pastime you've discovered lately. In any case, it's okay to be selfish sometimes. Place more focus on rejuvenation and you'll be happier and more effective during the day. Your family, your kids, whoever—they'll understand. In fact, they'll be glad you took the personal time to take care of yourself.

5. PURGE NEGATIVITY FROM YOUR LIFE.

There's no way around it. You must surround yourself with positivity if you want to accomplish great things. There can be no room in your life for negativity.

I realize more and more that our outlook, our attitude, what we think, and the words we speak influence everything around us. That's why I refuse to say bad things about other people, because negativity only breeds more negativity, diluting the quality of my thoughts, and consequently the quality of my life. I find positive, uplifting people to befriend, and I look for the good, rather than the bad, in people and situations.

Always remember how powerful it is to be positive. Pay attention to your thoughts. Watch the words you use, and notice how you say them. Stay focused on the positives, and allow that awesome attitude to bring you health, peace, joy, and fulfillment.

There's nothing standing in your way of a better life, apart from yourself. Build great habits and create the life you want. It's your decision.

And that, my friends, is the bottom line.
See you in the sunshine!

Stay Relentless!
Christmas

Scientific Bibliography

Abete, I., et al. 2008. Specific insulin sensitivity and leptin responses to a nutritional treatment of obesity via a combination of energy restriction and fatty fish intake. *Journal of Human Nutrition and Dietetics* 21:591–600.

Baer, D.J., et al. 2011. Whey protein but not soy protein supplementation alters body weight and composition in free-living overweight and obese adults. *The Journal of Nutrition* 141:1489–94.

Bassit, R.A., et al. 2000. The effect of BCAA supplementation upon the immune response of triathletes. *Medicine & Science in Sports & Exercise* 32:1214–19.

Canfi, A., et al. 2011. Effect of changes in the intake of weight of specific food groups on successful body weight loss during a multi-dietary strategy intervention trial. *Journal of the American College of Nutrition* 30:491–501.

Canoy, D., et al. 2005. Plasma ascorbic acid concentrations and fat distribution in 19,068 British men and women in the European Prospective Investigation into Cancer and Nutrition Norfolk cohort study. *American Journal of Clinical Nutrition* 82:1203–9.

De Palo, E.F., et al. 2001. Plasma lactate, GH, and GH-binding protein levels in exercise following BCAA supplementation in athletes. *Amino Acids* 20:1–11.

Dreher, M.L., and A.J. Davenport. 2013. Hass avocado composition and potential health effects. *Critical Reviews in Food Science and Nutrition* 53:738–50.

Faber, M. et al. 1986. Dietary intake, anthropometric measurements, and blood lipid values in weight training athletes (body builders). *International Journal of Sports Medicine* 7:342–46.

Flood-Obbagy, J.E., and B.J. Rolls. 2009. The effect of fruit in different forms on energy intake and satiety at a meal. *Appetite* 52:416–22.

Halton, T.L., and F.B. Hu. 2004. The effects of high protein diets on thermogenesis, satiety and weight loss: A critical review. *Journal of the American College of Nutrition* 23:373–85.

Hamid, R., et al. 2005. Beneficial metabolic effects of regular meal frequency on dietary thermogenesis, insulin sensitivity, and fasting lipid profiles in healthy obese women. *American Journal of Clinical Nutrition* 81:16–24.

Hassmen, P., et al. 1994. Branched-chain amino acid supplementation during 30-km competitive run: mood and cognitive performance. *Nutrition* 10:405–10.

Herron, K.L., et al. 2004. High intake of cholesterol results in less atherogenic low-density lipoprotein particles in men and women independent of response classification. *Metabolism* 53:823–30.

Hill, A.M., et al. 2007. Combining fish-oil supplements with regular aerobic exercise improves body composition and cardiovascular disease risk factors. *American Journal of Clinical Nutrition* 85:1267–74.

Iglay, H.B., et al. 2009. Moderately increased protein intake predominately from egg sources does not influence whole body, regional, or muscle composition responses to resistance training in older people. *Journal of Nutrition and Healthy Aging* 13:108–14.

Jailal, I., et al. 2013. Increased chemerin and decreased omentin-1 in both adipose tissue and plasma in nascent metabolic syndrome. *The Journal of Clinical Endocrinology and Metabolism* 98:E514–17.

Johnstone, A.M., et al. 2012. Safety and efficacy of high-protein diets for weight loss. *The Proceedings of the Nutrition Society* 71:339–49.

Layman, D.K., and D.A. Walker. 2006. Potential importance of leucine in treatment of obesity and the metabolic syndrome. *Journal of Nutrition* 136:319S–323S.

Mourier, A., et al. 1997. Combined effects of caloric restriction and branched-chain amino acid supplementation on body composition and exercise performance in elite wrestlers. *International Journal of Sports Medicine* 18:47–55.

Murphy, K.J., et al. 2012. Effects of eating fresh lean pork on cardiometabolic health parameters. *Nutrients* 4:711–23.

Nile, S.H., and S.W. Park. 2014. Edible berries: bioactive components and their effect on human health. *Nutrition* 30:134–44.

Panickar, K.S. 2013. Effects of dietary polyphenols on neuroregulatory factors and pathways that mediate food intake and energy regulation in obesity. *Molecular Nutrition & Food Research* 57:34–47.

Rebello, C.J., et al. 2013. Dietary strategies to increase satiety. *Advances in Food and Nutrition Research* 69:105–82.

Rossi, A.M., and B.E. Katz. 2014. A modern approach to the treatment of cellulite. *Dermatologic Clinics* 32:51–59.

Soares, M.J., et al. 2003. Is there a role for monounsaturated fat in the dietary management of obesity? *Asia-Pacific Journal of Public Health* 15 Supplement:S18–21.

Tipton, K.D., et al. 2003. Acute response of net muscle protein balance reflects 24-h balance after exercise and amino acid ingestion. *American Journal of Physiology, Endocrinology and Metabolism* 284:E76–89.

Vander Wal, J.S., et al. 2005. Short-term effect of eggs on satiety in overweight and obese subjects. *Journal of the American College of Nutrition* 24:510–15.

Wadden, T.A., et al. 2009. One-year weight losses in the Look AHEAD study: factors associated with success. *Obesity* 17:713–22.

White, P.J., and M.R. Broadley. 2009. Biofortification of crops with seven mineral elements often lacking in human diets—iron, zinc, copper, calcium, magnesium, selenium and iodine. *New Phytologist* 182: 49–84.

Xiao, Q., et al. 2013. A large prospective investigation of sleep duration, weight change, and obesity in the NIH-AARP Diet and Health Study cohort. *American Journal of Epidemiology* 178:1600–10.

Yang, Q. 2010. Gain weight by "going diet?" Artificial sweeteners and the neurobiology of sugar cravings: Neuroscience 2010. *The Yale Journal of Biology and Medicine* 83:101–8.

Yau, Y.H., and M.N. Potenza. 2013. Stress and eating behaviors. *Minerva Endocrinologia* 38:255–67.

Zemel, M.B., and X. Sun. 2008. Calcitriol and energy metabolism. *Nutrition Reviews* 66: S139–46.

Index